Your First ENT Job

A survivor's guide

Marie Lyons
ENT Registrar
North Thames Region

and

Arvind Singh
Specialist Registrar
Royal Marsden Hospital

T0372204

Foreword by

Ram Dhillon
Consultant in Otolaryngology
Northwick Park Hospital, Harrow

Radcliffe Publishing
Oxford • Seattle

Radcliffe Publishing Ltd
18 Marcham Road
Abingdon
Oxon OX14 1AA
United Kingdom

www.radcliffe-oxford.com
Electronic catalogue and worldwide online ordering facility.

© 2006 Marie Lyons and Arvind Singh

British Library Cataloguing in Publication Data

A catalogue record for this book is available from the British Library.

ISBN 1 85775 748 3

Typeset by Anne Joshua & Associates, Oxford
Printed and bound by TJ International Ltd, Padstow, Cornwall

Contents

Foreword

Hardly a month passes before further, and not always acceptable, changes need to be implemented by our medical and political masters in the training of clinicians and other non-medical staff. This has had the consequence of numerous additional subjects being added into time-constrained undergraduate medical training and a soon to be shortened framework at postgraduate level. This has already resulted in an inevitable ditching or severe curtailing of exposure to a number of specialties. ENT, amongst others such as dermatology, infectious diseases etc., has been such a victim.

Regulations such as the European Working Time Directive and policies such as Modernising Medical Careers have conspired to shorten the working week and the period of training. Perversely, the latter is likely to also result in more, but less experienced, clinicians encountering ENT during the foundation years.

The authors have been in the maelstrom of health change and have personal experience of the many problems alluded to above. This has facilitated their goal of providing a book that is concise, has a fluid style and highlights the essential practical aspects needed to work in ENT.

This melange of a backdrop provides the reason for the book's title, *Your First ENT Job: a survivor's guide*, as it fulfils a need for healthcare professionals who will encounter patients with ENT diseases. It should become a helpful addition to doctors in an ENT post but more specifically for individuals in

A&E, nurse practitioners and for those involved in cross-cover for ENT. Although a basic textbook in the subject, it introduces the day-to-day practicalities that are essential to delivering ENT care by providing the requisite level of clinical knowledge and its attached science.

Professor Ram Dhillon FRCS
Consultant ENT Surgeon, Northwick Park Hospital, Harrow
Honorary Professor, Middlesex University, London
September 2005

Preface

Welcome to ENT. We realise that you may feel a bit over-whelmed by the subject, especially as you possibly won't have had much exposure to it before. You also may not be working in ENT as your day job – you may be covering at night or even be an Accident and Emergency officer. We too were once new to ENT, and we remember the trepidation of our first few days. We decided to write this practical guide in a 'what to do when faced with X' format, as we think we would have found it very useful as new SHOs.

ENT can seem very daunting at first, as it is often inadequately covered at medical school. It is also a speciality where you will learn to perform many new procedures that you haven't seen before. Remember, however, that you are a doctor first, and please do not leave this knowledge at the door of the hospital! Resuscitation and ABC are just as valid, if not more so, in ENT. Common sense and a pragmatic, calm attitude are also helpful. Panic does neither you nor the patient any good. We have written this manual in an attempt to help you to cope before you start to panic.

We have also included a brief summary of the common ENT operations and what you must tell the patient and discuss with them. We have tried to be as comprehensive as possible, but inevitably there will be a few less common operations which we have omitted. If you have no idea what the operation involves, please ask someone before you consent the patient! If there is no one to ask at the time, leave the consent to someone more senior – it will be less stressful for both you and your patient.

ENT is a great speciality with plenty of variety in the types of patients and conditions that you treat. We hope you enjoy it.

Marie Lyons
Arvind Singh
September 2005

About the authors

Marie Lyons was born in Co. Limerick, Ireland, in 1972. She moved to London at the age of 14 years and attended secondary school before going up to Cambridge in 1990, winning the Tyer's scholarship. Having completed a degree in medical sciences she went on to clinical studies at Addenbrookes Hospital, Cambridge. After house jobs, she returned to London and joined the Chelsea & Westminster/Watford surgical rotation, where she completed the MRCS. She began ENT training as an SHO in 1999 and continues to work as an ENT registrar in the North Thames region. Marie lives in Hertfordshire with her husband and baby son.

Arvind Singh was born in 1972 in a small town in Greater London. He studied at his local sixth-form college before obtaining a place to study medicine at University College and Middlesex Schools of Medicine. He achieved a first-class honours intercalated degree in anatomy and neuroscience, funded by the Shanks scholarship. Following his medical degree he completed basic surgical training at Basildon Hospital. He began his otolaryngology training at Basildon Hospital and continued as an SHO at St Mary's Hospital and the Royal Free Hospital. He commenced higher surgical training in 2001 in the North Thames region. He is currently based at the Royal Marsden, where he is developing his expertise in head and neck oncology.

Marie Lyons

I would like to thank my husband Adam for all his help and support when we were writing this book. He was a wonderful unofficial editor, correcting my English and making the text more reader friendly (even for a lay person). I couldn't have done it without him. I would like to dedicate the book to my lovely boy Thomas who was born two days after I submitted the manuscript. He has certainly had early exposure to ENT!

Arvind Singh

I would like to thank my family for their immense support, and in particular my wife for her patience and understanding during all the late evenings spent working.

Ears

1 Ears

Basic anatomy

The external ear consists of the pinna and the outer ear canal (*see* Figure 1.1). The outer third of the ear canal is cartilaginous, hair-bearing and wax-producing. It is also not particularly sensitive, which makes it relatively easy to inspect with an auroscope. The inner third is bony and exquisitely sensitive. Push too deep into the bony ear canal and the patient will certainly protest! The outer ear canal ends at the eardrum, which in a healthy ear is a pale grey structure (*see* Figure 1.2). The most obvious features are the handle of the malleus and antero-inferiorly the cone of light (see below). When you are shown a picture of the eardrum you can always identify which side it is on by the direction in which the malleus is pointing. If the eardrum is on the right side, the malleus will point upwards and superiorly to the right from the middle of the eardrum. If it is on the left side, the malleus will point to the left (amaze your boss at quizzes!).

When looking at the eardrum you will see a cone of light. This is the part of the drum that is perpendicular to the light from the auroscope, and its position will change depending on the health of the eardrum. In a healthy drum it lies antero-inferiorly.

The eardrum is the lateral border of the middle ear, and some middle ear structures can occasionally be seen through it. The

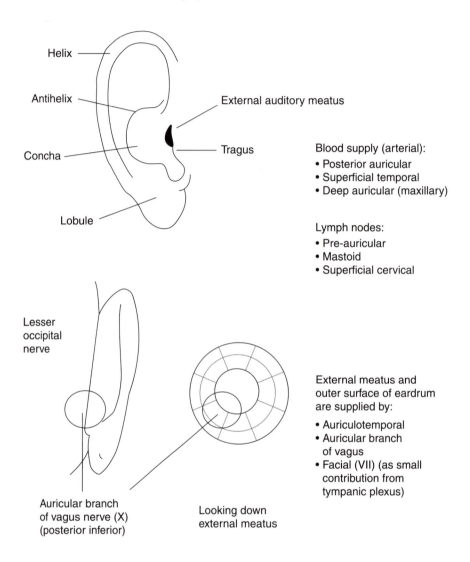

Ear – right pinna and external meatus

Helix

Antihelix

Concha

Lobule

External auditory meatus

Tragus

Blood supply (arterial):
• Posterior auricular
• Superficial temporal
• Deep auricular (maxillary)

Lymph nodes:
• Pre-auricular
• Mastoid
• Superficial cervical

Lesser occipital nerve

External meatus and outer surface of eardrum are supplied by:

• Auriculotemporal
• Auricular branch of vagus
• Facial (VII) (as small contribution from tympanic plexus)

Auricular branch of vagus nerve (X) (posterior inferior)

Looking down external meatus

Figure 1.1 View of outer ear canal and schematic view of eardrum.

Tympanic membrane
- Three layers
  - Inner – low columnar
  - Middle – fibrous
  - Outer – stratified squamous
- 1 cm diameter
- Pearly grey and shiny
- 55 degrees to horizontal
- Concave outwards
- Faces downwards, forwards and laterally
- Pulled inwards by tensor tympani
- Sensory supply
  - Inner – glossopharyngeal (IX)
  - Outer – auriculotemporal (Vc)
- Vibrates with oncoming sound
- Needs equal air pressure on
  each side of it (see auditory tube)

Viewed down an auroscope

Anterior   Posterior

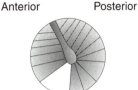

Cone of light
(antero-inferior)

**(a) View of tympanic
membrane from the
ear canal**

Middle ear – left tympanic membrane

Corda tympani
over pars flaccida

Posterior

Umbo

Pars tensa

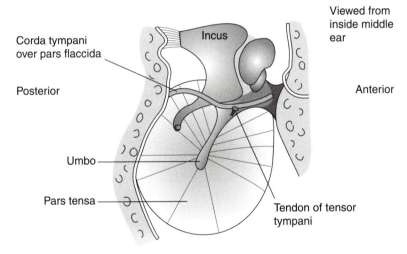

Incus

Viewed from
inside middle
ear

Anterior

Tendon of tensor
tympani

(b) View of tympanic membrane from the middle ear

Figure 1.2   View of middle ear.

most obvious structure is the malleus, as this is attached to the underside of the eardrum. Occasionally the incus can be seen tucked behind the malleus. Antero-inferiorly a white bulge can be seen. This is the promontory, which is the marker for the basal turn of the cochlea.

Box 1.1   More detailed anatomy of the ear

If you are a career ENT SHO or are interested please read on. We shall attempt to make the anatomy of the inner ear simple, so the following account will only scratch the surface (ENT registrars go on week-long courses in order to fully get to grips with the anatomy!). If you only want the basics feel free to skip this section, as you probably will not need to know it for day-to-day practice (although pathology may make more sense if you know the anatomy).

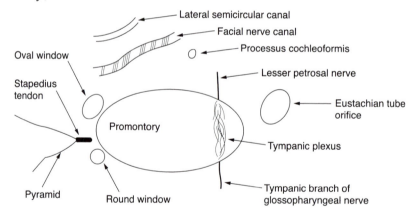

Figure 1.3 Medial wall of middle ear.

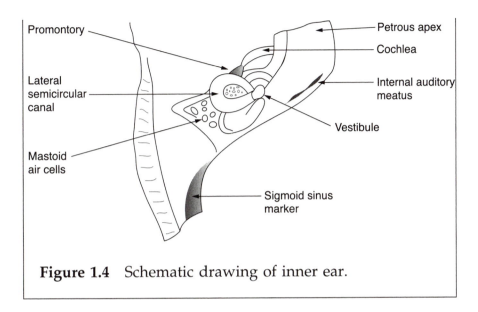

Figure 1.4 Schematic drawing of inner ear.

Facial nerve

The facial nerve is included in this section as its anatomy is both complicated and intimately related to the middle and inner ears. A knowledge of its anatomy will allow you to determine whether an injury to the facial nerve (e.g. as a result of a skull fracture) is likely to be temporary and the various ways in which you can assess the level of injury.

Intracranial part

The facial nerve has mixed sensory, motor and secretomotor fibres and special sense (taste) fibres. The facial nerve proper contains motor fibres (supplying the muscles of facial expression), with the rest being included in the nervus intermedius which accompanies the facial nerve for part of its course.

The facial nerve nucleus lies in the caudal part of the pons, and it loops around the abducens nucleus in the floor of the fourth ventricle. It emerges at the lower border of the pons with the nervus intermedius, and both travel to the internal auditory meatus along with the vestibulocochlear nerve. The facial nerve enters its bony canal above the vestibule of the labyrinth. At the first genu lies the geniculate ganglion, and the greater petrosal nerve leaves the main facial nerve at this point to supply the nasal and lacrimal glands. Taste fibres from the palate relay impulses in the opposite direction. The facial nerve proper turns posteriorly at this point, and the outline of its canal can be seen between the promontory and the lateral semicircular canal (*see* Figure 1.3). Some branches leave the nerve at this point and join the tympanic plexus. The nerve eventually turns again, this time inferiorly medial to the aditus ad antrum to reach the stylomastoid foramen. The corda tympani leaves the facial

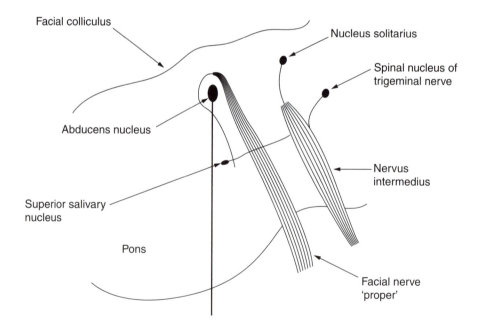

nerve about 5–6 mm above the stylomastoid foramen to enter the middle ear. It runs over the pars flaccida between the malleus and the incus. It passes out of the middle ear anteriorly at the tympanic notch. It emerges from the petrotympanic fissure along the medial part of the spine of sphenoid and joins the lingual nerve. The corda tympani carries taste fibres from the anterior two-thirds of the tongue and secretomotor fibres to the floor-of-mouth salivary glands.

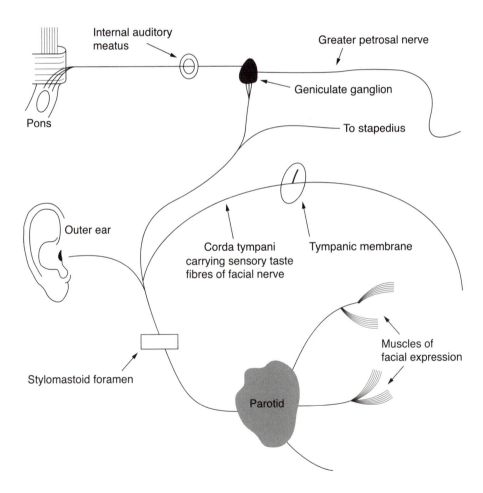

Figure 1.6   Schematic drawing of the facial nerve (2).

Extracranial part

Once it emerges from the stylomastoid foramen, the facial nerve is embedded in parotid tissue. It usually divides into upper and lower divisions and it has five terminal branches (temporal, zygomatic, buccal, mandibular and cervical).

Questions you need to ask about ear problems

- Is the ear painful? If so, what is the nature and site of the pain?
- Is the ear itchy?
- Is there discharge? If so, describe the amount, consistency, colour and smell.
- Is there hearing loss?
- Is there tinnitus (noise in the ears, which can be subjective or objective)? If so, what is its nature (constant/intermittent/pulsatile)?
- Is there vertigo (an illusion of movement)?

Examination of hearing using tuning-fork tests

This seems to cause confusion, but Table 1.1 should clarify matters. Basically you are trying to ascertain whether the ear is better at conducting through air (normal) or through bone (abnormal).

Rinne's test is performed by making a 512 Hz tuning fork resonate and then placing it on the mastoid process (this tests bone conduction). The patient is asked whether they can hear

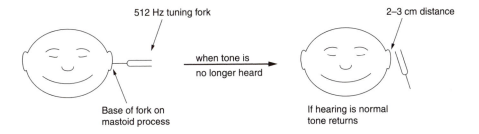

Figure 1.7   Rinne's test.

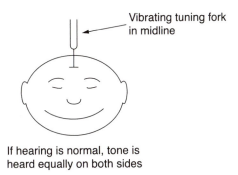

Figure 1.8   Weber's test.

Table 1.1 The meaning of the results of Rinne's test and Weber's test

Rinne's test	Weber's test	Result
Positive (air better than bone)	Central	Normal hearing
Positive	To unaffected ear	Sensorineural hearing loss
Negative (bone better than ear)	To affected ear	Conductive loss
Negative (false)	To unaffected ear	Profound loss or 'dead ear'

the noise of the tuning fork and to report when the noise dies away. The tuning fork is then placed 2 cm away from an unobstructed ear canal (*see* Figure 1.7) and the patient is asked whether they can still hear it (this tests air conduction). (A normal positive result occurs when air conduction is better than bone conduction.)

Weber's test is used to determine whether there is better hearing in one ear than in the other. A resonating tuning fork is placed on the midline of the forehead and the patient is asked first whether they can hear the tone, and secondly whether they can hear it better on one side. A normal result occurs when the tone can be heard equally well on both sides.

How to deal with ear problems

We shall deal with the conditions you will commonly encounter, from lateral to medial location.

Pinna (including pre-auricular area)

The most commonly seen conditions are probably trauma and infection.

Trauma

This can be sharp or blunt. Your first priority is always maintenance of a safe **A**irway, ensuring that the patient is **B**reathing and taking steps to maintain the **C**irculation. Ascertain the mechanism of injury (remember that head injuries take priority, as these are much more likely to be fatal).

Inspect the ear and its surroundings. Examine the outer ear canal, and also examine the facial nerve and document its function.

Sharp object trauma

- This is usually fairly easy to deal with. Under local anaesthesia repair the skin of the pinna. The skin should be approximated (but not too tightly) to prevent haematoma collection. Try to repair the skin only and not to put the stitches through the cartilage.

- Give the patient antibiotics and review them in clinic the next day.

- If there is very severe injury or the ear has been removed completely, plastic surgery intervention may be necessary unless the ENT consultant has wide experience in facial plastics.

Blunt injury

- The main feature to look for is a *pinna haematoma*. Once you have seen one you won't forget it! It is a boggy, often bluish swelling which obscures the normal contours of the ear. The danger with this type of injury is that if left it can become infected and cause cartilage destruction, leading to a cauliflower ear (*see* Figure 1.9). It must therefore be drained immediately.

- **Do not leave it until the emergency clinic the next day!**

- Initially a pinna haematoma can be *aspirated under local anaesthesia. Apply a pressure dressing and give antibiotics.* A pressure dressing consists of a non-adhesive dressing with an ear shape cut out of it, gauze, a large wedge of cotton wool and a firmly applied elastic bandage.

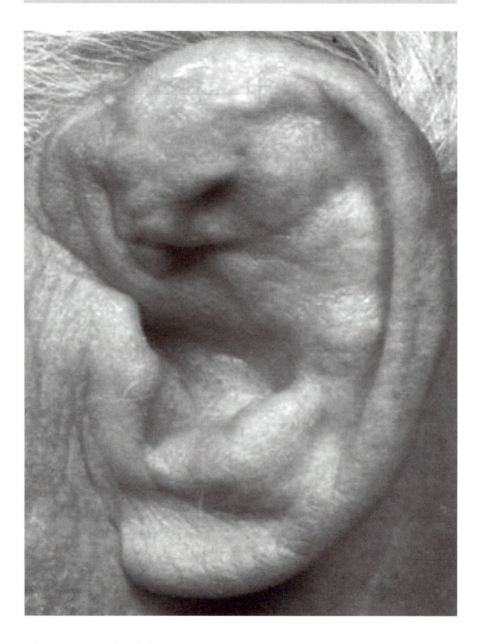

Figure 1.9   Cauliflower ear.

- *Review the next day.* If the haematoma has not re-collected, the patient can be sent home and reviewed in two days' time (although they must return sooner if there is an increase in pain or swelling). If it has re-collected, the patient will require definitive management in theatre. (Ask the patient to come for review starved just in case.)

Infection of the pinna

- Often this is an extension of otitis externa. The pinna is painful, red, hot and swollen.

- If the infection is very severe the patient may need admission for intravenous antibiotics.

- Always make a point of asking if the patient is diabetic, as the infection tends to be much more serious in such cases. It is often worth obtaining a random blood sugar monitoring even if the patient is not a known diabetic.

Pre-auricular sinus

- The ear develops from six hillocks of mesenchyme, so it is not surprising that congenital abnormalities occur. One of the commonest is a pre-auricular sinus where two of the hillocks do not fuse properly. It is visible as a small pit in front of the superior part of the helix.

- Nothing needs to be done about a pre-auricular sinus unless it becomes infected. If it is merely red with no abscess then it may settle with antibiotics, but an appointment must be made to review the patient.

- If there is an abscess, the patient will require incision and drainage.

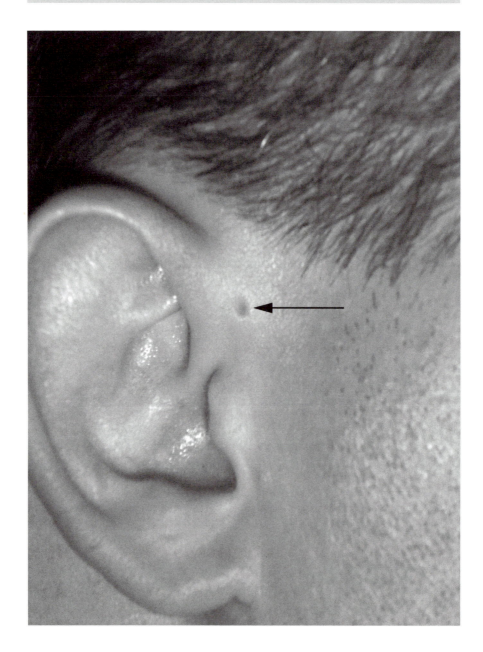

Figure 1.10   Preauricular sinus.

- If the patient has recurrent infections then the sinus should be excised, but the patient should be warned that it is sometimes very difficult to excise it altogether and there is a possibility of the sinus recurring.

Outer ear canal

The commonest referrals are for foreign bodies in the ear, infection and trauma.

Foreign body

- This is very common in children.

- Unless the foreign body is a caustic substance it can be seen in the next available clinic slot.

- Always examine the patient under the microscope and not just with an auroscope, as it is easy to miss foreign bodies with the latter.

- If the object is smooth and round it is better to get a hook behind it and flick it out rather than using forceps, which may push it further in. Paper, sponge or similar materials can be eased out with suction or crocodile forceps.

- *Make just one attempt, especially with children or uncooperative adults.*

- If you cannot remove the object, list the patient for general anaesthetic removal (this is preferable to causing trauma to the ear canal or eardrum).

- Reassure the patient that the foreign body will do no harm (provided that it is an inert material) if left for a few days. However, vegetable matter (e.g. a pea) needs to be removed as soon as possible as it can swell and cause extreme ear pain.

- Insects can be drowned with water before removal.

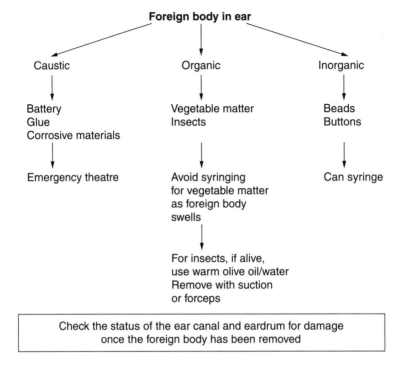

Figure 1.11 How to deal with a foreign body in the ear.

Infection

There seems to be much confusion about the difference between the terms otitis externa and otitis media. *Otitis externa,* as the name suggests, is inflammation of the outer ear canal. It is painful, and moving the pinna exacerbates the pain. There is discharge but it tends to be scanty. Gentle examination (and you would be well advised to be gentle!) reveals a red swollen outer ear canal. However, you cannot be sure that it is just otitis externa if you cannot see the eardrum, as otitis media with a perforation and profuse discharge can also cause secondary otitis externa.

The treatment of otitis externa is topical. As much debris as possible should be cleaned out under the microscope. Take a swab and remember to ask for a fungal culture, especially if the GP has already used drops. If the ear canal is open, give eardrops (Sofradex or Gentisone) and review the patient in the clinic in a week or so. If the ear canal is very narrow or closed, insert a wick. Either use a pope wick (which, like a tampon, expands lengthways and widthways to open up the ear canal) to give the drops, or else use ribbon gauze soaked in bismuth iodoform paraffin paste (BIPP) or Tri-Adcortyl ointment. There is no need for eardrops with a BIPP or Tri-Adcortyl wick. We tend to prefer a pope wick (*see* Figure 1.12) because it expands and can also be placed in a single motion (never underestimate exactly how painful this condition is!). The patient must keep their ear meticulously dry, especially when washing their hair. Tell them to put cotton wool covered in Vaseline into the concha before showering. They need to be reviewed in two to three days for removal and replacement of the wick if necessary. Warn the patient that insertion of the wick is painful but that the pain should ease once the wick is in place.

Again, remember to ask if the patient is diabetic. If they are and the pain seems to be out of proportion to the appearance of the ear, they probably require admission for intravenous antibiotics (ciprofloxacin) and control of blood sugars as they may have malignant otitis externa, which leads to osteitis of the temporal bone. A CT scan may be necessary to confirm the diagnosis. Malignant otitis should be taken very seriously indeed, as it has a significant morbidity and even mortality associated with it.

Otitis externa: summary

- Inflammation of the outer ear.

- Movement of the pinna is painful.

- Treatment is topical after suction clearance (drops and/or wick).

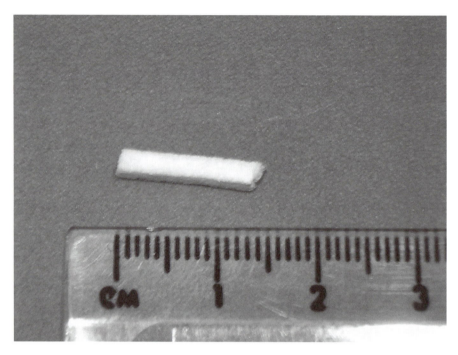

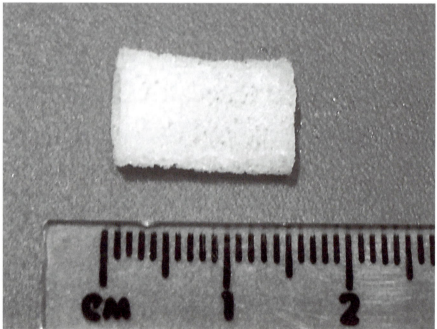

Figure 1.12 (a) Pope wick; (b) expanded pope wick.

- The ear should be kept dry.

- Remember diabetes, and be alert for malignant otitis externa.

Acute otitis media

As the name suggests, this is inflammation of the middle ear. It is a painful condition, but touching the pinna does not usually exacerbate the pain, which is caused by pressure on the ear-drum. The onset of discharge usually relieves the pain. The discharge is much more copious and also thinner than that of otitis externa.

On examination the ear canal appears normal (unless there is superimposed otitis externa), but the eardrum is red and can be bulging. There may be a perforation, in which case you should document its position and size (*see* Figure 1.13).

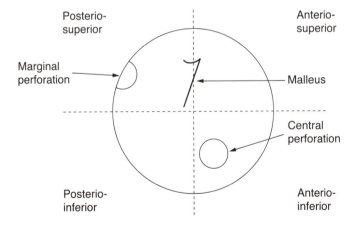

Figure 1.13   Positions on tympanic membrane and central and marginal perforations.

You also need to document whether the perforation is central (i.e. you can see drum all round the perforation) or marginal (in which case the hole extends to the edge of the eardrum). A marginal perforation is more suggestive of deeper disease (e.g. underlying mastoid disease or cholesteatoma).

The treatment is systemic with oral antibiotics and review.

Remember that with any ear disease it is important to obtain an audiogram as soon as possible. All patients should have an audiogram before they are discharged from the clinic. If the ear canal is 'closed' because of otitis externa, wait until it has opened before requesting an audiogram. If you send a patient for an audiogram with a large amount of discharge in the ear, don't be surprised if you get a rude note back from your audiologist and no audiogram – they *always* look in the ear before they do their tests. Let them know in advance and try to remove as much discharge as possible – you will get a much better result. Never send a patient with discharge for a tympanogram, as the discharge will contaminate the probes.

Otitis media: summary

- Inflammation of the middle ear.

- Movement of the pinna does not exacerbate the pain (unless there is superimposed otitis externa).

- There is a copious runny discharge (pain is often relieved by the onset of discharge).

- Hearing is decreased and there may be perforation of the eardrum.

- Treatment is systemic.

- Remember to look behind the ear for inflammation (consider the possibility of mastoiditis).

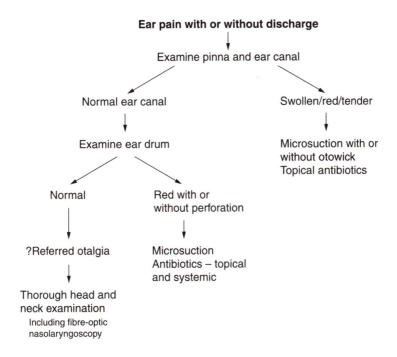

Ear pain with or without discharge

Examine pinna and ear canal

Normal ear canal   Swollen/red/tender

Examine ear drum   Microsuction with or without otowick Topical antibiotics

Normal   Red with or without perforation

?Referred otalgia   Microsuction Antibiotics – topical and systemic

Thorough head and neck examination Including fibre-optic nasolaryngoscopy

Figure 1.14 How to deal with ear pain: summary.

Mastoiditis

This usually occurs as a consequence of otitis media. The area behind the pinna is red and tender when touched. The ear is usually pushed forward to give an asymmetrical 'bat ear'. Assess the status of the patient (are they showing signs of meningitis?), admit them for intravenous antibiotics and inform a senior colleague. Try to assess the patient's hearing with tuning-fork tests (there is usually a conductive loss). Assess and document facial nerve function. A CT scan may be necessary (go down to radiology and ask for fine cuts of the temporal bone). If there is some concern about the possibility of meningitis, a CT head scan and neurosurgical opinion may be necessary. If there is an abscess, it may require incision and drainage in theatre with or without a cortical mastoidectomy and grommet insertion.

Outer ear canal trauma

Trauma to the outer ear canal may be due to sharp objects or blunt trauma and skull fractures.

- Injury to the outer ear canal caused by a sharp object can usually be treated conservatively by giving antibiotic drops and keeping the ear dry. Trauma to the eardrum can also be treated conservatively, but a baseline-hearing test should be performed initially and the patient should be reviewed after a few weeks.

- Trauma to the middle and inner ears usually results from a head injury. *Remember that it is the head injury that could kill the patient and this takes priority.* Examine the ear carefully and look for eardrum perforations, haemotympanum (blood behind the eardrum) and facial nerve palsy. If there is a possibility of a skull base fracture, speak to a radiologist and discuss obtaining special fine cuts on a CT scan of the skull base, as a CT head scan is not adequate (radiologists appreciate people asking their advice and trying to involve them in the case).

- Immediate ENT surgical intervention is usually only under-taken if there is acute total facial nerve palsy after head injury with a proven skull base fracture, and the suggestion that there may be a fragment of bone leading to paralysis.

Temporal bone fractures

Temporal bone fractures are classified according to their orientation relative to the axis of the temporal bone. The two main types are transverse and longitudinal (*see* Figure 1.15).

In practice, fractures are rarely truly one type or the other, but usually a combination of both. Transverse fractures tend to go across the facial nerve (usually at the level of the labyrinth),

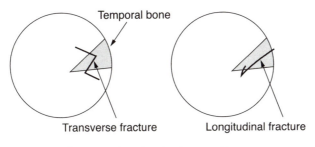

Cross-section showing temporal bone

Figure 1.15 Schematic diagram showing transverse and long-itudinal temporal bone fractures.

and paralysis is more likely to be permanent. Longitudinal fractures sometimes lead to damage to the facial nerve, usually at the level of the geniculate ganglion. Deafness occurs due to different mechanisms for each type of fracture. Longitudinal fractures lead to conductive deafness by causing bleeding into the middle ear or ossicular dislocation. Transverse fractures may disrupt the vestibulocochlear nerve, and deafness is much more likely to be permanent.

Miscellaneous conditions of the ear and surrounding structures

Sudden-onset sensorineural deafness

Take a history and examine the ear, looking for infection, perforation and vesicles. Examine the facial nerve (especially if vesicles are present in the ear canal). Perform Rinne's and Weber's tests to assess whether the deafness is conductive (in which case Rinne's test will be negative and Weber's test will show 'better' hearing on the affected side) or sensorineural (in which case Rinne's test will be positive and Weber's test will show 'better' hearing on the unaffected side). If the deafness is sensorineural, admit the patient for carbogen treatment (5% CO_2 in 95% O_2 for 5 minutes every hour for 24 or 48 hours, but check your hospital's policy), and give steroids (prednisolone 40 mg dose for 1 week, but again check local policy as your consultant may have another regime) and acyclovir (this is usually a standard dose of 800 mg five times a day). Obtain a formal hearing test as soon as possible. An urgent MRI scan will probably be required the next day. If the deafness is conductive then the patient can be sent home if seen out of hours, but they should be seen again the next day to have a formal hearing test to confirm the diagnosis. If the deafness is of several days' or weeks' duration, the above medications are less likely to work. However, it is worth leaving the choice up to the patient, as they may want to try treatment in the hope that it will be of some benefit. Those who recover quickly are likely to have the best outcome.

Sensorineural hearing loss: summary

- History and examination (Rinne's test and Weber's test).
- Causes may include a viral cause or summary vasoconstriction of an end artery.
- Treatment consists of steroids, acyclovir and vasodilators (carbogen, dextran). The effectiveness of these treatments has not been proven beyond all doubt.
- MRI scan.

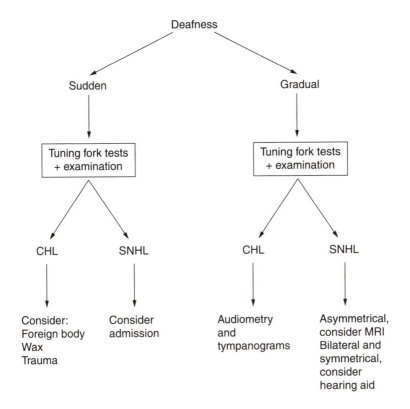

Figure 1.16 How to deal with deafness. CHL, conductive hearing loss; SNHL, sensorineural hearing loss.

Facial nerve palsy

- This presents to ENT because of the possible need for surgical intervention.

- Examine the ear for signs of infection or vesicles, and perform a full neurological examination (this may be a cerebrovascular accident). ENT facial palsy is usually total and a lower motor neuron lesion (i.e. there is no forehead sparing).

- If the ear appears normal or has vesicles and the rest of the neurology is normal, treat with steroids and acyclovir. If the patient is seen in the daytime, get a hearing test and also assess stapedial reflexes (this gives an indication of the level of the palsy; *see* Figure 1.6).

- *The eye is the most important structure to protect in a patient with facial nerve palsy.* Give the patient antibiotic eye ointment and instructions on how to tape the eye shut (an eye patch is insufficient, and a cotton-wool patch over the eye may lead to abrasion of the cornea if the eye is not closed first). They should be referred to the eye clinic for assessment (get some idea of function by examining the eye yourself first, before you refer the patient). If you do experience problems getting the patient seen, this is a situation in which you must be quite firm and insistent. Remember that you are responsible for the patient until they are seen by the team to whom you have referred them. 'The team refused to see the patient' is not a great defence.

If the ear appears abnormal with infection, admit the patient for intravenous antibiotics and steroids. They may need surgical decompression of the nerve. Speak to someone senior and consider obtaining a scan of the temporal bone (this may show facial canal dehiscence).

You must document severity of disability. This should include ability to close the eye (complete, partial or none) plus facial asymmetry (at rest or on movement). Alternatively you could use the House–Brackmann grading system (*see* Table 1.2).

Dizziness

- This is seen more commonly in the ENT clinic, but the occasional dizzy patient is referred from Accident and Emergency.

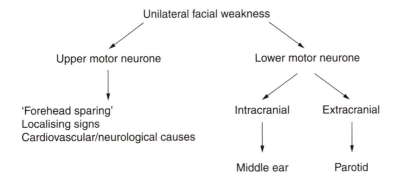

Figure 1.17 How to deal with facial nerve palsy.

Table 1.2 House–Brackmann scale

Grade	Description	Measurement*	Function (%)	Estimated function (%)
I	Normal	8/8	100	100
II	Slight paralysis	7/8	76–99	80
III	Moderate paralysis	5–6/8	51–75	60
IV	Moderately severe paralysis	3–4/8	26–50	40
V	Severe paralysis	1–2/8	1–25	20
VI	Total paralysis	0/8	0	0

*This denotes the superior movement of the mid portion of the superior eyebrow and lateral movement of the oral commisure.

The score is one point for every 2.5 mm of movement of each component up to 10 mm. The points are added together and a maximum score of 8 can be obtained if each structure moves by 10 mm.

- A good history is the most important factor in the care of these patients. They can be notoriously vague, so it is important to pin down the exact details of the dizziness. For example, is it vertigo (an illusion of movement) or light-headedness? When did it start? What was the patient doing? Did they feel sick? Did they fall over? How long did the dizziness last? Was there a change in hearing or tinnitus?

- It is also vital to take a *full* medical history, including a list of drugs taken (both prescribed and over the counter).

- The patient must have a full examination, including a full neurological examination. If they are so unsteady that they cannot walk and they live on their own, they probably need admission and prescription of Stemetil and possibly betahistine. An audiogram should be performed as soon as possible (the next day if the patient is seen after hours).

Table 1.3 Dizziness patterns and possible causes

	BPPV	*Ménière's disease*	*Labyrinthitis*	*CP angle lesion*
Onset	Sudden	Sudden	Sudden	Sudden (if acute bleed into lesion) or gradual
Lasts	Seconds to minutes	Minutes to hours	Hours to days	Progressive, ongoing
Nausea	Mild	Yes, can be severe	Yes	Yes
Relation to movement	Yes	No	No	Can occur

BPPV, benign postural positional vertigo; CP, cerebropontine angle.

- Consider an urgent MRI if the dizziness is not settling. One of the authors remembers being caught out by a patient who had all the signs and symptoms of benign positional vertigo. As matters didn't improve, an MRI was arranged and an acoustic neuroma was found.

Preparing patients for ear surgery

Specific points to remember include the following.

- Remember to take a history and ask if there are still problems. In children, for instance, glue ear is a transient condition and may well have resolved while the patient is on the waiting list.

- Examine the ear, and if it is full of wax this should be removed if possible (not every pre-admission clinic has all of the facilities necessary – just do your best). If you see infection, start treatment (although for mastoid surgery this is probably not necessary). Remember that many surgeons will not perform a myringoplasty on an infected ear.

- Read through the notes and if a scan has been done make sure that it will be available for the day of operation. (In an ideal world it should be available at pre-admission and you should look at it in order to inform yourself about the case). You should make it your responsibility to ensure that all scans are present for the list you will be attending (getting on the right side of a good ward clerk is essential here).

- *All* patients who are having ear surgery will need a hearing test within the three months prior to surgery.

- If cosmetic operations are to be performed on the ear (e.g. pinnaplasty), photographs will also be needed.

Ear operations

Foreign body removal

This involves examination of the ear under the microscope and removal of the foreign body. This is usually straightforward with no ill effects. However, there may sometimes be a small amount of bleeding for a few hours after the operation if the removal was difficult. Very rarely the drum may be damaged by the insertion or removal of the foreign body. This should heal spontaneously if the ear is kept dry and possibly some antibiotics are given. *Always* consent to look in both ears, especially if you are operating on a small child. They are very good at putting objects in both ears, and you will look pretty silly if you miss it. It is important to look at both ears under the microscope, as you can miss a foreign body when examining a wriggling child with an auroscope.

Grommet insertion (see Figure 1.18)

This involves examining the ear under the microscope, removing any wax and debris and making a tiny hole in the eardrum with a special knife. Any fluid in the middle ear is sucked away. It is impossible to remove all of the fluid, but enough is removed to ease the insertion of the grommet; the rest will disappear within a few days. A small ventilation tube called a grommet is then placed through the hole in the eardrum (like a button through a buttonhole). This allows 'fresh' air into the middle ear and prevents the glue from forming.

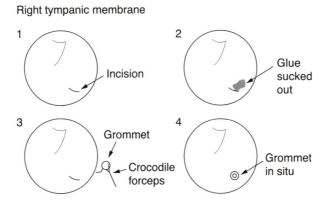

Right tympanic membrane

Figure 1.18   Grommet insertion.

Risks of the procedure

- In many children there is a little bleeding and/or discharge for a few days afterwards. This is normal and nothing to be too alarmed about. The surgeon will decide at operation whether antibiotic drops should be given for a few days after the surgery.

- Grommet insertion is a temporary measure to allow time for a child to recover from glue ear naturally. The grommet stays in for 6 to 12 months and usually comes out on its own. Very occasionally a grommet needs to be removed if it has been in place for over two years.

- Once the grommet has extruded the problem will usually settle, but glue ear can recur, especially if the child was very young at first insertion. More than one set of grommets may be necessary, and it is difficult to predict which child will need more than one set.

- If the child has had grommets inserted for recurring infections, they can still get infections with the grommets *in situ*. However, these tend to be painless infections. The ear must be protected from water, especially dirty or soapy water.

- Usually once the grommet has extruded the eardrum heals spontaneously (the healing drum pushes the grommet out). However, in about 10% of patients the perforation does not heal. The perforation is observed for up to a year to give it a chance to heal, and it can be repaired at a later date. It is preferable to wait until a child is more mature before repairing a quiescent perforation, in order to reduce the likelihood of a recurrent glue ear.

Pinnaplasty (see Figure 1.19)

This is an operation to correct prominent or 'bat' ears. These usually occur because the antihelix fold of cartilage has not formed properly. It is usually performed in children for cosmetic reasons and to stop them being teased/bullied at school. An incision is made behind the ear and sometimes excess skin is removed. A new fold of cartilage is formed by stitching with permanent (silk) sutures, scoring or drilling the cartilage. Sometimes the conchal bowl is sutured down to the mastoid periosteum. A firm head bandage is then applied and worn for 1 week post-operatively. This is then removed in clinic and a headband (a sports headband will suffice) should be worn at night for 6 weeks. 'Before' photographs must be taken and should be available in the notes at the operation.

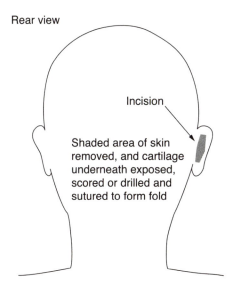

Rear view

Incision

Shaded area of skin
removed, and cartilage
underneath exposed,
scored or drilled and
sutured to form fold

Figure 1.19   Pinnaplasty.

Risks of the procedure

- Bleeding/haematoma, as the pinna has a rich blood supply. Usually bleeding during the operation is not too much of a problem and the surgeon makes sure that the pinna is dry before finishing the operation. A pressure bandage also makes haematoma formation less likely. Occasionally a haematoma can form. If there is an increase in pain and throbbing of the ear after operation, the patient should probably return to hospital to have the pressure bandage removed and the ear inspected. Any haematoma will need to be drained (possibly in theatre in the case of young children) with antibiotic cover.

- Infection. Antibiotics are given by some surgeons, but nevertheless infection can occur. This is treated with a broad-spectrum antibiotic.

- Suture failure and failure of correction of abnormality. Sometimes a stitch can disintegrate and the antihelical fold can unfold. This is less likely to occur if the scoring or drilling methods are used. If the cosmetic result is not acceptable the operation may need to be repeated.

Myringoplasty (see Figure 1.20)

This is an operation to repair an eardrum perforation. The approach depends on the site and size of the perforation. The first part of the operation involves preparation of the edges of the perforation ('freshening') **(a)**. This involves scratching the edges of the perforation and getting back to healing eardrum tissue. Tiny perforations in ears with wide canals can be repaired using a fat patch harvested from the lobule of the ear. They are repaired permeatally. Larger or more inaccessible

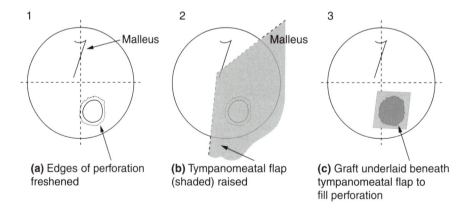

(a) Edges of perforation freshened

(b) Tympanomeatal flap (shaded) raised

(c) Graft underlaid beneath tympanomeatal flap to fill perforation

Figure 1.20   Myringoplasty.

perforations are repaired using temporalis fascia harvested via an endaural or postaural incision. A tympanomeatal flap (eardrum plus ear canal skin) is raised **(b)** and the graft is placed underneath the eardrum **(c)**.

Risks of the procedure

- If an external approach is used, there will be an endaural or postaural scar. This is not usually noticeable once it has healed, but always ask about keloid scarring. If the patient is prone to keloid scarring, obtain consent for injection of the wound site with steroid as this may help prevent the development of keloid scars.

- Failure rates are around 10–15%. Even if the perforation does not heal completely, it usually ends up smaller. Failure rates for repeat operations are higher than for the initial operations.

- 'Dead ear' or decreased hearing: This is unusual but can possibly occur due to injury to middle ear structures. Always warn the patient that the purpose of a myringoplasty is to give a clean dry safe ear and not to improve hearing. If the hearing improves then this is an added bonus.

- Dizziness. This is usually temporary and settles after a few days.

- Taste disturbance. The corda tympani runs very close to the eardrum, and it is often necessary to disturb it in order to place the graft. This leads to a metallic taste on the operated side of the tongue. This will settle but may take several months to do so, especially if it was necessary to divide the nerve in order to place the graft.

- Tinnitus. This is usually temporary but it may persist.

Mastoid surgery

Mastoid surgery involves exploring the middle ear and mastoid air-cell system, and removing chronic infection to yield a safe dry ear. The incision is endaural or postaural and involves lifting a tympanomeatal flap. It also involves drilling the mastoid to remove unhealthy tissue. It is one of the more major ear operations.

Risks of the procedure

- Scarring (as for myringoplasty). If an external approach is used, there will be an endaural or postaural scar. This is not usually noticeable once it has healed, but always ask about keloid scarring. If the patient is prone to keloid scarring, obtain consent for injection of the wound site with steroid as this may help prevent the development of keloid scars.

- Head bandage and ear packing. The bandage stays on for 24 hours and the packing remains for up to 4 weeks.

- 'Dead ear' or reduction in hearing. Dead ear results from damage caused to internal ear structures by drill noise. The more usual scenario is a reduction in hearing because the ear disease involved some of the ossicles, which therefore had to be removed. Sometimes the cholesteatoma itself conducts sound, and its removal will therefore lead to a discontinuity in the sound conduction pathway. If this is the case, reconstruction may be possible once the chronic infection has been eradicated.

- Facial nerve damage. As mentioned in the anatomy section above, the facial nerve is intimately related to the middle ear and mastoid antrum. Great care is taken to identify the facial nerve, but damage can still occur. It is essential to demonstrate what a facial nerve palsy looks like and to make sure that the patient understands. You should also stress that there are remedial measures which can be taken to correct the damage, but these will take several months to work.

- Dizziness. Many patients who have undergone middle ear surgery feel dizzy for a few days afterwards. This usually resolves spontaneously.

- Tinnitus. Patients who have had mastoid surgery usually have packing in the ear which remains *in situ* for up to 3 weeks. This itself can cause tinnitus. However, tinnitus may persist after removal of the packing.

- Recurrence. Chronic ear infection can be difficult to eradicate, and sometimes a repeat operation is necessary. If a canal wall-up procedure is carried out the patient will need a 'second-look' operation in 12 to 18 months' time to look for recurrence.

Stapedectomy

This operation is performed in cases of otosclerosis, a condition that causes fixation of the ossicles, especially the stapes. Initially the hearing loss is conductive, but later on cochlear sclerosis can lead to sensorineural deafness. It is diagnosed on the basis of history and examination (clinically the eardrum will look normal in most cases, although there may be increased redness over the promontory). Rinne's test is negative in the affected ear, and Weber's test shows a response in the affected ear. The audiogram shows a conductive hearing loss with Cahart's notch at 2000 Hz (*see* Figure 1.21).

Tympanograms are normal or slightly reduced in amplitude on the affected side, and the stapedial reflex is reduced or absent on the affected side. A stapedectomy is performed permeatally, and a tympanomeatal flap is raised. A small

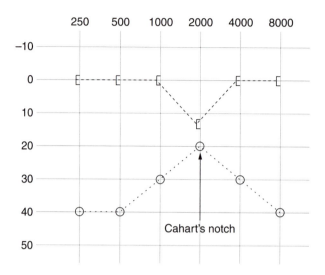

Figure 1.21 Audiogram showing otosclerosis of right ear with Cahart's notch.

part of the posterior canal wall is removed. The stapedius tendon is divided and the stapes is removed. A hole is made in the footplate (using laser or a microdrill) and a stapes prosthesis is placed between the incus and the footplate. Most of the pistons are made of Teflon. The eardrum is then replaced and gelfoam is placed in the ear canal.

Risks of the procedure

* Failure to perform the operation. The diagnosis should always be checked once the middle ear has been opened. Congenital abnormalities of the other ossicles can also cause conductive deafness. If the stapes is not fixed then the procedure is abandoned. Sometimes the anatomy of the middle ear and the facial nerve will not allow the procedure to be performed without damage to other structures, in which case again the procedure may be abandoned.

- 'Dead ear' due to endolymph leakage.

- Facial nerve damage. The facial nerve runs just above the footplate and must be protected when laser is used. The procedure is abandoned if it cannot be performed without causing facial nerve damage.

- Dizziness. Many patients are dizzy postoperatively, and some have nystagmus. This usually settles spontaneously.

- Displacement or extrusion of the prosthesis. This can happen early or late. The only treatment is a hearing aid or re-operation.

- Taste disturbance. This is the same as for any exploration of the middle ear.

- Tinnitus. This is a common feature of otosclerosis. Surgery usually helps tinnitus, but it can persist or even worsen after operation.

Neuro-otological procedures

These are very complex and often involve collaboration between neurosurgery and ENT. Unless you are very experienced and have read up on these procedures, it is probably best to leave the consenting to someone more senior (remember to tell your senior colleague that you have done this).

Nose

2 Nose

Basic anatomy

The nose is a pyramidal structure formed from bone and cartilage. It is divided into two nares (nostrils) by the septum, which itself consists of bony and cartilaginous parts. Each nostril has a floor, a roof, a straight medial wall and a sloping lateral wall. The posterior part opens into the nasopharynx via a posterior choanae. The floor of the nose is formed by the palate, mainly the hard palate (this is why it is always vital to look in the mouth when examining the nose, as the floor of the nose is the roof of the mouth). The roof is formed from the cribiform plate and is pierced by the olfactory nerve. This is why it is necessary to sniff in order to smell things properly, as doing so allows olfactory epithelium to be exposed to odour 'molecules'. The lateral walls consist of nasal mucosa covering tiny bones called conchae or turbinates. These increase the surface area of the nose and allow the air to be warmed and moistened on inhalation. The edge of the nostril also has hairs (vibrissae) that trap dust. The nose is very well supplied with blood vessels from both the external and internal carotid systems. The external carotid system supplies blood mainly via the sphenopalatine branch of the maxillary artery. There are also branches from the labial artery. The anterior ethmoidal artery is a branch of the internal artery, and is the artery that is sometimes damaged in nasal fractures.

Nasal cavity boundaries and coronal view

- Nasal cavity extends from nares to choanae
- Floor: hard palate
- Roof: sphenoid and ethmoid
- Medial wall: septum
- Lateral wall: medial orbit, ethmoidal air cells, maxillary sinus

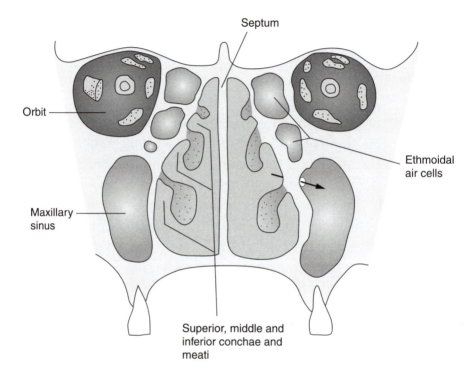

Mucosa:
- Olfactory nerve
- Vestibular – skin and hair
- Respiratory – pseudostratified
            ciliated columnar

Figure 2.1   Basic anatomy of the nose.

Nasal septum

Bones and
blood
supply

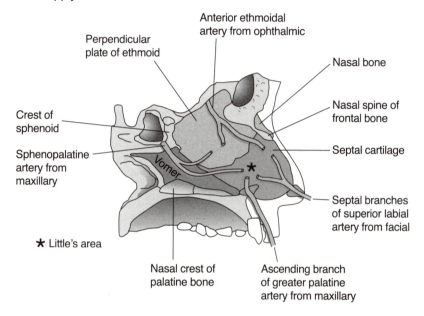

Perpendicular
plate of ethmoid

Anterior ethmoidal
artery from ophthalmic

Nasal bone

Nasal spine of
frontal bone

Crest of
sphenoid

Sphenopalatine
artery from
maxillary

Vomer

Septal cartilage

Septal branches
of superior labial
artery from facial

★ Little's area

Nasal crest of
palatine bone

Ascending branch
of greater palatine
artery from maxillary

Venous drainage
- Anterior – to face
- Posterior – to pterygoid plexus. Also via ethmoidal veins to ophthalmic and
  inferior cerebral veins; 1% via foramen caecum to superior sagittal sinus

Lymphatic drainage
- Lateral wall and septum. Posterior: to retropharyngeal and to anterior/superior
  deep cervical. Anterior: to submandibular

Lining
- Respiratory epithelium – pseudostratified ciliated columnar
  with mucous cells and very vascular
- Olfactory epithelium – ciliated nerve cells, yellowish, on
  roof and septum, under superior concha and in
  spheno-ethmoidal recess

Figure 2.2 View of medial part of the nose.

Questions you need to ask about nasal problems

- Is the nose blocked? If so, on which side is it blocked and is this constant?

- Is the sense of smell decreased or absent?

- Is the sense of taste decreased or absent?

- Is there rhinorrhoea? If so, what colour is the discharge and is it bloodstained?

- Is there postnasal drip? If so, what colour is it and is it bloodstained? Can the patient actually feel mucus dripping down the back of the throat or does it seem like a lump?

- Is there facial discomfort (often a feeling of pressure or heaviness which gets worse on leaning over)?

How to deal with nasal problems

Epistaxis

There is a misconception that epistaxis is a trivial condition. However, *it is serious and potentially life-threatening*. The nose bleeds because it has a very rich blood supply from both the external and internal carotid systems (*see* Figure 2.2). These anastomose at Little's area, at the antero-inferior end of the septum. This is the most common site of bleeding in children. In adults the situation tends to be slightly more complicated.

- When faced with an epistaxis, the basic principles of treatment of shock apply, namely to stop the bleeding and resuscitate the patient. Get a *large* line in (the absolute minimum is green, but bigger is better). Take blood samples for a full blood count and clotting G&S as a minimum. Also do urea and electrolytes if the patient is on medication, and possibly liver function tests if there is a suggestion of alcohol abuse.

- Next you must *stop the bleeding*. Basic first aid is to pinch the *soft* part of the nose just below the nasal bones and sit the patient upright (if their conscious level allows) so that they can spit out any blood. Ice often helps. Remember to protect your face, eyes and clothes with a mask, goggles and apron (there will be blood going everywhere and you don't want it in your eye!).

- Always ask a member of nursing staff to help you, and don't take the patient to a room far away from everyone else, as fainting often occurs, especially if packing is necessary.

- If the bleeding is not very severe, soak some cotton wool in cophenylcaine (a combination of local anaesthetic and vaso-constrictor), put it in the affected nostril and leave it for a few minutes. A useful trick is then to push the cotton wool back with a sucker until a bleeding point appears, which can then be cauterised. We tend to use silver nitrate. Don't aim the cautery stick directly at the bleeding point or you will start the epistaxis again. Cauterise the area around the bleeding point first, and then move on to it. If the epistaxis stops, keep the patient in the department for at least an hour to make sure that it doesn't start again. If the patient is a frail elderly person with no support at home and it is late, consider admission.

- If you cannot stop the bleeding or it is very severe, packing the nose is probably necessary. Merocel is a first-line pack. Anaesthetise the nose (packing really hurts!) and use the largest pack available, as small ones are fairly ineffective. Remember that the nose goes *backwards* toward the neck and not upwards towards the top of the head. Push the pack along the floor of the nose firmly and as quickly as you can. *Hesitating will make it worse for the patient.*

- In our opinion all patients with packs should be admitted, and this is also the policy at many hospitals that have an on-site ENT service. Other hospitals may have different policies. The patient needs to be observed closely. Antibiotics should be given and also possibly sedation with low-dose diazepam (2 mg three times a day) (but beware the frail elderly person with chest problems).

- If Merocel does not work, the next pack to try is BIPP, which is kept in the fridge. It is supplied as a long ribbon soaked in antiseptic. Hold the free end of the BIPP and using Tilleys dressing forceps push a length along the floor of the nose as far as you can. Then get another length of ribbon and layer this over the first one. Always leave the free end extending

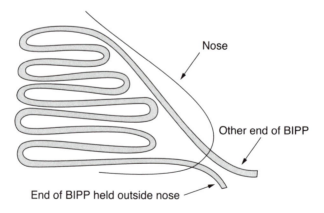

Figure 2.3 How to place BIPP.

out of the nose, as otherwise it will migrate into the patient's throat. Put in as much as you can fit.

• If this doesn't work, you may need a postnasal pack. Some hospitals have epistat catheters, but if all else fails, a Foley catheter will suffice. We have found that the best way to insert a Foley catheter is to push it along the floor of the nose and observe the throat until the catheter tip just appears behind the soft palate. Then pull it back by about 0.5 cm and inflate the balloon with *air* (there is a risk of aspiration if water or saline is used). You then need to pull the catheter forward until it stops moving forward and seems to be sitting snugly on the postnasal space. The catheter is then held in position using an umbilical clamp. *Always* protect the ala of the nose from the clamp with a lyofoam dressing. You will also need to pack the front of the nose after inserting a catheter. Epistat catheters have an anterior balloon which will do this for you.

• If the bleeding still won't stop, then it's time to get help.

• **If the bleeding occurs after nasal trauma, be especially vigilant. These tend to be the most catastrophic life-threatening bleeds. They need careful observation and early intervention.**

Foreign body in the nose

This problem is quite common, especially in children. Try to spray their nose and inspect it. As described for ears in the previous chapter, if the foreign body is smooth or round it is better to get a hook behind it and flick it out along the floor of the nose. If it is paper you can use a crocodile forceps. All foreign bodies in the nose that cannot be removed under local anaesthetic require admission and removal as quickly as possible, as there is a risk of aspiration. The only possible exception is the child who has had unilateral smelly discharge for weeks or months, as they are highly unlikely to aspirate the foreign body if it has been present for so long. Obviously, however, it is desirable to remove it as soon as possible, as school can be a pretty unpleasant place for these children.

If a child comes to the emergency clinic with unilateral epistaxis and/or foul-smelling discharge, consider the possibility of a foreign body. There is less risk of aspiration associated with these 'old' foreign bodies, but nevertheless they should be removed as quickly as possible. Be especially careful with watch batteries. These constitute a surgical emergency and must be removed as quickly as possible because they leak and the contents are very corrosive to the lining of the nose.

Fractured nose

If the patient is well and there is no epistaxis and no *septal haematoma* (a boggy swelling of the septum which is usually seen bilaterally), they can be sent home. They should be reviewed in 5 days' time for assessment of the injury and discussion of whether the patient wants a manipulation under anaesthetic (MUA). If a septal haematoma is present the patient must have this drained (in theatre) as soon as possible in order to prevent infection and subsequent destruction of the septal cartilage, which leads to saddle deformity of the nose.

Acute sinusitis

The symptoms are a blocked nose, rhinorrhoea (although not in all cases), fever and facial pain which is well localised to the area over the sinuses. On examination, there may be some pus in the nose and there will certainly be tenderness over the sinuses. If the patient is unwell it is probably wise to admit them and treat them with intravenous antibiotics (a cephalosporin and metronidazole, as the infection may well be due to anaerobes), nasal decongestants and analgesia. Sinus X-rays are probably of little benefit, but a CT scan may be considered if the problem does not improve.

Periorbital cellulitis

- At first glance it may seem very odd that this is an ENT problem, but it is usually caused by sinusitis, and if surgical intervention is necessary, the ENT team generally undertakes it. Ideally, care of the patient is shared by ENT, ophthalmology and, in the case of children, paediatricians.

- The patient complains of a painful eye (which can be so swollen that it is shut) and may or may not have nasal symptoms. On examination the eye is red and swollen and there may be some proptosis.

- You *must* look at the eye (this sometimes requires prising the eye open) and assess colour vision and visual acuity (this is often difficult in a child, which is why it is mandatory to get an ophthalmology opinion urgently). *If the sight is threatened, colour vision is the first part of vision to deteriorate.* A note should also be made of the level of consciousness and a neurological examination should be performed, as the patient may develop cavernous sinus thrombosis, which can be fatal. The rest of the cranial nerves should be examined and documented (especially the abducens).

- The patient must be admitted for treatment with intravenous antibiotics and nasal decongestants, and eye observations should be performed regularly. Remember that if visual acuity starts to decline there is a very short window in which to save the sight.

- A CT scan will be necessary to assess the sinuses and to look for the presence of a subperiosteal abscess.

Cheek swelling

This is often referred to ENT, as we tend to be more commonly available than maxillofacial surgeons. In rare cases cheek swelling may be caused by sinus malignancy, but more often than not the cause is dental. This is no excuse for not examining the patient properly, and a full ENT examination (including nasendoscopy) should be performed. If you want to look really impressive you should do a basic examination of the teeth, as the carious one is usually obvious. Tapping the teeth will elicit pain if there is any decay. Obtain an orthopantomogram. If this is normal it may be worth getting a sinus X-ray, especially if the patient has worked with hardwoods, as these individuals are more prone to sinus malignancies.

Preparing patients for nasal surgery

For general considerations, *see* page 102. Most nasal operations involve correcting the structure of the nose (e.g. rhinoplasty, septoplasty) or operations on the sinuses. Except for septoplasty, most patients awaiting nasal operations will have had scans or photographs taken. You will be very unpopular with your boss and the patient if these are not available. If there is any doubt as to whether they have been obtained, ask the patient, as this is much more reliable than ringing round every outlying hospital searching for scans!

Nasal operations

Manipulation under anaesthetic (MUA)

This operation is done for a fractured nose with displacement. It involves giving a short general anaesthetic and literally pushing the nose straight again. It is done 10–14 days post injury. An external splint is placed if the reduced fracture is thought to be unstable. The splint stays on for 4–5 days and is made of aluminium or plaster of Paris

Risks of the procedure

- Bleeding. This sometimes occurs but usually settles spontaneously without packing.

- Imperfect result. The nose will probably not return to its pre-injury state. A septorhinoplasty may be necessary at a later date if the patient is unhappy with the appearance of the nose.

- Persistent septal deviation. MUA is primarily a cosmetic operation. If there has been concomitant septal fracture, MUA will not cure this. A septoplasty may be necessary at a later date if the deviation is symptomatic.

Foreign body removal

This is often performed under general anaesthetic in small children and uncooperative adults. The foreign body is removed using forceps or a hook, and you should consent to look at both sides of the nose while the patient is under anaesthetic.

Risks of the procedure

- The nasal mucosa is often friable when it has been exposed to a foreign body for a long time, and it often bleeds once the foreign body has been removed. This usually settles spontaneously.

- There may be damage to the nasal mucosa caused by a corrosive foreign body (e.g. watch battery) – adhesions can occur later.

Adenoidectomy

This involves removing adenoidal tissue. It is done through the mouth so there are no cuts or stitches on the outside. A tonsillectomy gag is put in the mouth and opened. The adenoids are felt and the palate can also be examined to rule out a submucosal cleft palate which is a relative contra-indication to adenoidectomy, especially if done using suction diathermy. If the adenoids are large or obstructive they are removed using a specially designed curette or removed by suction diathermy under direct vision. If the adenoids are small and non-obstructive they are not removed.

Risks of the procedure

- Bleeding. About 1 in 100 cases need to return to theatre.

- Regrowth. This can occur, but the adenoids do not usually become obstructive.

- Nasopharyngeal regurgitation. This is usually temporary while the soft palate 'learns' to close off the now wider nasopharynx.

Septoplasty

This operation is performed in order to straighten a bent septum that is causing nasal obstruction. It is done by incising the nasal mucosa, lifting the nasal mucosa, perichondrium and periosteum off the septum, and removing or straightening (e.g. via scoring) any bent cartilage and removing any bony spurs (*see* Figures 2.4 and 2.5). As the septum forms part of the supporting structure of the nose, it is vital that a keystone area of cartilage is preserved (*see* marked area in Figure 2.5).

Risks of the procedure

- Not curative. Many patients with nasal obstruction have a combination of rhinitis and septal deviation. If rhinitis is present, a septoplasty will not cure the symptoms completely. The degree of improvement will depend on the balance of obstruction caused by septal deviation and that caused by obstruction. However, a septoplasty may make taking medication for rhinitis easier.

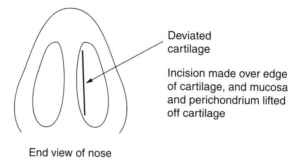

Deviated
cartilage

Incision made over edge
of cartilage, and mucosa
and perichondrium lifted
off cartilage

End view of nose

Figure 2.4 Septoplasty (1).

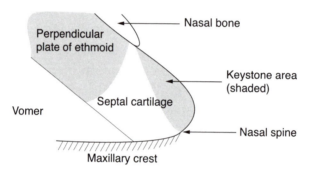

Nasal bone

Perpendicular
plate of ethmoid

Keystone area
(shaded)

Septal cartilage

Vomer

Nasal spine

Maxillary crest

Figure 2.5 Septoplasty (2).

- Bleeding. Many surgeons pack the nose after this operation, and the packs stay in for a variable length of time. The patient will have bloodstained mucous rhinorrhoea for up to 10 days after the operation. This is normal and not something to be alarmed about. If fresh bleeding occurs then the patient should return to hospital and may need fresh packing. Blood can also collect between the flap and the cartilage, causing a septal haematoma. If the patient experiences acute pain and the nose becomes completely blocked, they should return to hospital for assessment. A septal haematoma should be drained as soon as possible under antibiotic cover to prevent permanent cartilage damage.

- Blockage. It is very important to tell the patient that they won't feel better straight away and that they will feel as if they have a severe head cold for a couple of weeks after the surgery. It can take up to several months for the condition to settle completely.

- Numb teeth. Sometimes a septoplasty involves removing some of the maxillary crest which is deviated. This leads to numbness of the incisors which can take several weeks to settle.

- Septal perforation. Every care is taken to preserve the mucoperichondrial flaps while performing a septoplasty. With very sharp severe spurs this is sometimes impossible. However, it is usually possible to preserve the mucosa on one side. Occasionally a septal perforation (communication between the two nares via the septum) forms. It can cause crusting and dryness of the nose and lead to whistling on breathing in. It can be treated conservatively with cream and nasal douche, with a septal button. Operative repair is often very difficult.

- Saddle deformity. Even where every effort has been made to preserve the keystone area of tip support, a saddle deformity can still occur. This is supratip depression with some widening of the nasal bridge and some tip retraction. Correction can be difficult and would involve a rhinoplasty.

Rhinoplasty

This is an operation performed in order to change the external appearance of the nose. It is often combined with a septoplasty. The most important aspect of this operation is pre-operative preparation. The surgeon and the patient should have a full and frank discussion of the perceived problem, the patient's expectations and what is achievable. If there is any suggestion of psychological overlay, a psychiatric opinion should be sought. The patient must have pre-operative photographs. The operation is performed either internally (via an incision just in front of the nasal cartilage) or externally (via an incision on the columellar skin, but remember to warn about the scar, although it is barely visible once healed). There may also be stab incisions on the lateral part of the nose which are made in order to introduce osteotomes for fracture of the nasal bones if this is necessary.

Risks of the procedure

- Bleeding/bruising. Most patients have nasal packs for a variable length of time postoperatively. Almost all patients have periorbital bruising. Warn the patient that they will look terrible at first and that it will take several weeks for all the swelling to settle, and only then will the true result of the operation be evident.

- Nasal blockage (as for septoplasty).

- Imperfect result. This is why there must be a full discussion of the possibilities before the operation is performed.

Sinus surgery

For the most part this means endoscopic sinus surgery, although it also includes antral washouts and simple polypectomies. These are performed either by direct vision using a headlight (for washouts and polypectomies) or by using an endoscope. In both cases they are done through the nose and there are no cuts or stitches on the outside. Occasionally a septoplasty is necessary in order to gain access to the nose, and you should consent all patients who are undergoing endoscopic surgery for a septoplasty after explaining why it may be needed.

Polyps are removed, and generally endoscopic surgery involves uncinectomy and opening of the middle meatus. The anterior ethmoids are then opened and sometimes the posterior ethmoids, depending on the severity and extent of disease.

Due to the complicated anatomy of the sinus system, all endoscopic surgery will require prior scanning. These scans must be available for the surgeon. Many surgeons will not perform even simple polypectomy without a scan.

Risks of the procedure

- Bleeding. As for any nasal surgery.

- Nasal blockage postoperatively. As for all nasal surgery.

- Orbital damage. The ethmoidal complex lies very close to the eye. This is why scanning is so important, as it will alert the surgeon to abnormal anatomy. The lamina papyracea of the eye is extremely thin and easily breached. This is not a major disaster so long as it is recognised and the operation is finished at this point. This is also why any polyps that are removed are placed in saline, as polyps sink but orbital fat does not.

- Cerebrospinal fluid leakage. The ethmoid sinuses are also close to the cribriform plate, and a scan will reveal whether the cribriform plate is low-lying.

- Not curative. Unfortunately, even endoscopic sinus surgery cannot be guaranteed to cure sinus disease, especially polyps. Medical treatment may still be necessary, as may repeat procedures.

Procedures to stop epistaxis

If a decision is made to take a patient to theatre for epistaxis, the condition is generally fairly severe. The patient needs to be consented for all the procedures to stop epistaxis. These are as follows:

- inspection and simple cautery

- postnasal packing

- sphenopalatine ligation or diathermy

- maxillary artery ligation (endoscopically)

- anterior ethmoidal artery ligation (external approach)

- external carotid artery ligation in the neck.

Risks of the procedures

- Bleeding restarting postoperatively.

- ITU admission if a postnasal pack is placed.

- For endoscopic procedures, all the risks of endoscopic sinus surgery.

- Blood transfusion with all its inherent risks (infection, incompatibility, lowering of immune response).

- Scar and drain (for carotid artery ligation).

- Damage to nerves (IX and X) after carotid artery ligation.

Throat

3   Throat

Basic anatomy

See Figures 3.1 to 3.4.

Questions you need to ask about throat problems

- Is there pain? If so, where is it? Is there earache?

- Is swallowing affected? If there is a problem with swallowing, is it progressive and worse for solids or liquids?

- Are there problems with breathing?

- Does the patient make a noise when breathing?

- Are they or have they been a smoker?

We shall deal with the emergencies in order of how daunting they are to cope with. Airway problems are stressful even when you are more senior. We will give you tips on what to do reflexively, which will enable you to start to help the patient and will calm both of you down while help is on its way.

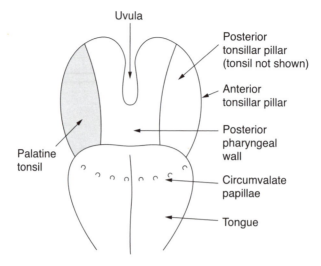

Figure 3.1   Anterior view of the throat viewed through the mouth.

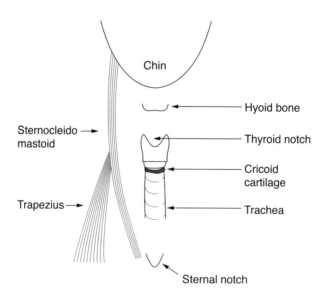

Figure 3.2   Schematic diagram of neck and important midline structures.

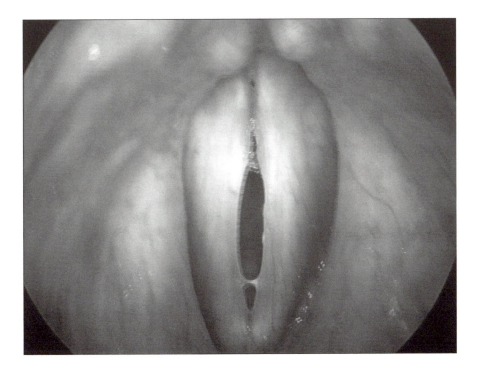

Figure 3.3 Normal larynx.

How to deal with throat problems

Supraglottitis/epiglottitis and stridor

Stridor is the term given to the harsh shrill sound of breathing through an obstructed airway. The more musical expiratory noise is termed wheeze. It is not a diagnosis in itself, and has many causes. If it is of sudden onset in a child, always think of a foreign body. Other causes include infection, tumours and vocal cord palsies.

Fortunately, since the introduction of haemophilus vaccine, epiglottitis has become very rare. The history is of a child who is unwell for a few days before presentation with a progressive sore throat. They will be sitting up drooling and breathing

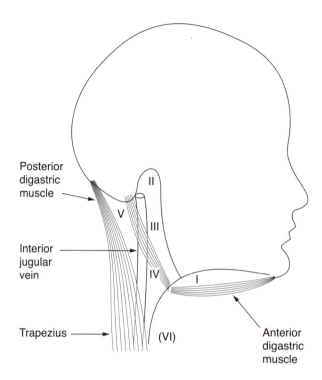

Posterior
digastric
muscle

II

V

III

Interior
jugular
vein

IV

I

Trapezius

(VI)

Anterior
digastric
muscle

Figure 3.4 Neck landmarks (surface anatomy and node levels). I, submental/submandibular region; II, along internal jugular vein from skull base to carotid bifurcation; III, along internal jugular vein from carotid bifurcation to omohyoid; IV, along internal jugular vein from omohyoid to clavicle; V, posterior triangle; VI, anterior compartment.

noisily (stridor), and they will also have a hoarse 'hot potato' voice. Call an anaesthetist and a registrar straight away. Do not do anything that will upset the child, and especially *do not try to look in their mouth!* You might try to waft an adrenaline nebuliser near the child's face, but only if it will not cause them to cry, as this may precipitate total airway obstruction. They should only be examined when a senior anaesthetist and ENT surgeon are present and prepared to intervene to secure the airway. The child should be intubated if at all possible and treated with antibiotics and steroids. A tracheostomy may be necessary, but it is a last resort.

Adults now present more commonly with supraglottitis. The history is similar to that of a child with epiglottitis. However, adults have more reserve, and treatment should be initiated immediately with adrenaline nebuliser (1 ml 1:1000 adrenaline with 4 ml saline), 8 mg dexamethasone (or 200 mg hydrocortisone) and intravenous antibiotics. Heliox (helium and oxygen) should be given, or if it is unavailable humidified oxygen should be given instead. The patient's airway can be assessed by flexible nasendoscopy. We often don't spray the nose with anaesthetic before we do the endoscopy, as we have found that the taste of the anaesthetic often makes the patient panic. If you feel that you will do a more efficient scope with anaesthetic, you should use it. Again you should call an anaesthetist and your registrar.

If the patient does not improve after the first nebuliser, give a second or even a third one. The patient may need intubation or even a surgical airway if there is no improvement. If they are severely ill, make sure that there is a tracheostomy set to hand. Ideally these patients should be admitted to a high-dependency unit, but at the very minimum they should be in a ward that is experienced in dealing with airway problems. They must be watched carefully.

Beware the 'tonsillitis' that has normal-looking tonsils, especially if there is a change in voice. All such patients should undergo nasendoscopy to make sure that they do not have supraglottitis.

When faced with a patient with supraglottitis, **CALL FOR HELP** while all the steps below are being prepared/executed.

- Nebulised adrenaline (1 ml 1:1000 in 4 ml saline)

- 8 mg dexamethasone IV

- Antibiotics IV

- Humidified O_2 or heliox if available

How to perform a cricothyroidotomy

This is one of the occasions when you will literally save a patient's life within the time it takes to place a definitive airway.

The cricoid cartilage is the easiest cartilage to palpate in the neck. The cricothyroid membrane lies above it, between the cricoid and thyroid cartilages. Find this and stay in the midline. If a cricothyroid needle is not available, use the largest venflon you can find and attach a syringe. Go straight down in the midline, and aspirate once you think you have reached the tracheal lumen. Then attach the needle/venflon to a three-way

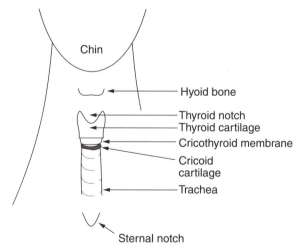

Figure 3.5   Cricothyroidotomy (*see also* Figure 3.2).

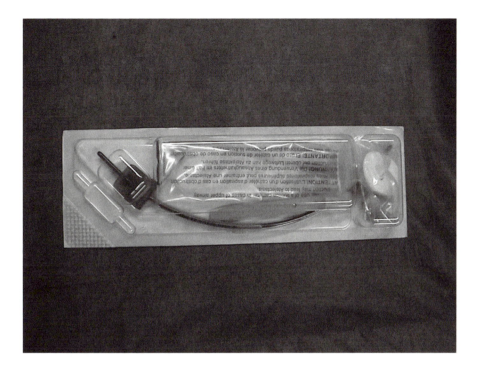

Figure 3.6 Cricothyrotomy set.

tap and connect it to an oxygen supply. You can 'jet' ventilate the patient by this method until more senior help arrives.

The greatest obstacle to performing this procedure is hesitancy on your part. Just remember that you have the ability to save the patient's life, even though taking an instrument to someone's neck is very daunting!

Tracheostomy

Most ENT surgeons will go straight to a tracheostomy when faced with an airway in jeopardy, rather than performing a cricothyroidotomy. This has the advantage that the airway is

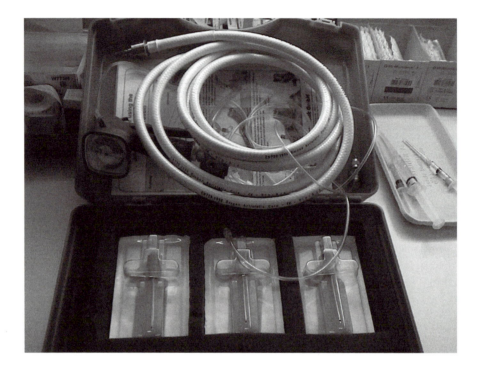

Figure 3.7 Jet insufflation kit.

secured definitively, and tracheostomy can be performed very quickly if necessary.

The classical teaching is to make a vertical incision for an emergency tracheostomy (your incision choice will depend on your experience; more experienced surgeons who have done many elective tracheostomies use the conventional horizontal incision). Hold the trachea steady with your non-dominant hand, and with your dominant hand make an incision in the midline below the cricoid cartilage. Make a reasonably long incision (there will be no prizes for cosmesis here!). You should be able to reach the trachea in two strokes of the knife (remember to stay in the midline). When you make an incision into the trachea there will often be a hiss of escaping air. You can then put your finger in the trachea and guide a tube into it.

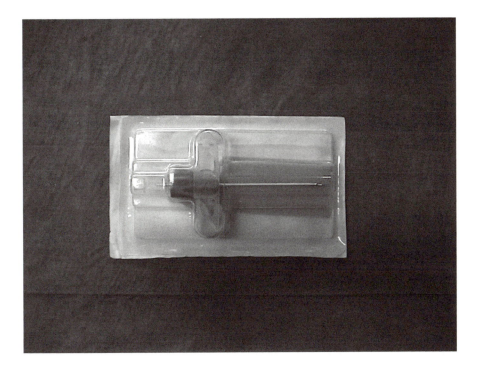

Figure 3.8 Transtracheal catheter.

You sometimes have to take the patient to theatre to stop any bleeding and tidy up the wound, but the main thing is that you have a secure airway (make sure that you hold on to the tube while the patient is being transferred).

Care of a tracheostomy

A clear airway is a human's most vital and precious possession, and a tracheostomy is nothing to be frightened of. If properly cared for it is very safe, and many patients manage their own tracheostomies for many years with little trouble. However, the complications and potential problems should be borne in mind, and every effort should be made to minimise them.

Immediate complications

- Bleeding. This can be minimised by a good knowledge of neck anatomy and always taking time to assess exactly where you are in the neck in relation to the trachea. In general you need to stay in or near the midline (remembering that the trachea may not always be a midline structure). Take time to stop and feel whether you are dissecting on to trachea and not wandering off to the side.

- Pneumothorax/haemothorax. This can occur if you are dissecting deep in a short neck.

- Damage to thoracic duct. Assessing and reassessing your position as described above for minimising bleeding will reduce the risk.

Early complications

All patients need close observation post tracheostomy (ideally they should be 'specialed' by a member of staff experienced in looking after tracheostomies). *On no account should they be put in a side room alone on a non-surgical ward.*

- Cardiac arrest. Many patients who undergo tracheostomies have chronically obstructed airways, and the sudden relief of this can cause problems. This is why they must be closely monitored after the operation.

- Dislodged tracheostomy: Tracheostomy tubes should be stitched in place at the end of the procedure and secured with tapes. Great care should be taken to hold the tube in place while moving the patient. The most important thing is to recognise when a tube has become displaced (the tube appears to be in an abnormal position, oxygen saturation levels drop or swelling develops in the neck) and to call for help early.

- Surgical emphysema. There is a small leak around all tracheostomies, even with cuffed tubes. It is important not to suture the wound too tightly around the tracheostomy tube, as the leaking air may be forced into the surrounding tissues (surgical emphysema). If surgical emphysema does develop, always bear in mind that the tube may have become displaced. It is often safer to call an anaesthetist and reintubate the patient rather than struggle with a tube that has become displaced. Once the patient is intubated you will have plenty of time to replace the tracheostomy tube in a calm controlled manner.

- Blocked tube. If at all possible, tracheostomy tubes with inner tubes are used, as the inner tube can be removed for easy cleaning. Initially a patient with a tracheostomy needs very regular suction (you cannot put a definite time on it, as the amount of suction needed varies from patient to patient). Regular suction and humidification of oxygen will prevent blockage.

Late complications

- Subglottic stenosis. This can be prevented by placing the tube below the second ring of the trachea.
- There may be a poor scar if the patient is prone to keloid scarring.

Ludwig's angina

- This is inflammation of the floor of the mouth. It can be serious because it pushes the tongue upwards and can result in blockage of the airway.

- It presents as swelling and pain in the floor of the mouth and dysphagia. On examination, look for neck swelling and look inside the mouth, noting the position of the tongue and whether there is stridor.

- All patients are admitted for intravenous antibiotics, steroids, analgesia and rehydration. If there is any doubt about the airway, an anaesthetist should be called and the airway secured either by intubation or by tracheostomy insertion.

Post-tonsillectomy bleeding

- This is usually mild but can be catastrophic. There are two peaks of incidence. The first is within 24 hours after operation, and the second is between a week and 10 days after the operation. The patient may just cough or spit up a small amount of blood, or they may bleed profusely. In the authors' opinion, these patients should all be admitted and given antibiotics.

- As with any bleeding patient, it is important to obtain good intravenous access and send blood for a full blood count, clotting and group and save. If the bleeding has stopped, admit the patient and give them antibiotics and mouthwashes (hydrogen peroxide if this is available), especially if there is a clot in the tonsillar fossa. Some authors advocate removing the clot by suction. However, we often find that this starts the bleeding off again. Another approach is to cauterise the area with silver nitrate, which occasionally works. If the bleeding has stopped, it is probably wise just to leave everything undisturbed. If the throat looks completely dry and the history is of a mild bleed, you can probably allow the patient fluids. Bear in mind that if the bleeding does start again the patient will need a 'crash' induction anyway, as some blood will have been swallowed. If the patient is at all unstable, keep them nil by mouth.

• If the bleeding continues and you have a co-operative patient, it is worth removing any clots by suction and holding cotton wool or a swab soaked in adrenaline and local anaesthetic over the area. This will often stop the bleeding.

• If you can't stop the bleeding, call for senior ENT help, call an anaesthetist and warn theatre.

Neck injuries

These can either be caused by sharp objects (e.g. knives, bullets, glass) or they may be blunt injuries (e.g. near hanging, attempted strangulation).

Injury by sharp objects

Assess the patient's airway and breathing (remember that the dome of the lung can be injured by a stab wound to the neck). Assess the cranial nerves (trigeminal, facial, glossopharyngeal, vagus, accessory and hypoglossal, depending on the site of the injury). Enquire about haemoptysis and haematemesis. Examine the patient for surgical emphysema (the air in the tissues will crackle like an air-filled sponge when palpated). All but the most superficial injuries (superficial to platysma in the entire length) probably need to be explored in theatre. Call for senior help, obtain a chest X-ray and intravenous access, and send off blood samples for a full blood count, clotting and cross-matching. You should also warn theatre and the anaesthetist.

Blunt injury

This may not seem very serious initially, but the danger is the later development of oedema and airway compromise. All such patients should be admitted and be given intravenous anti-biotics, steroids and possibly heliox. A flexible nasendoscopy should be performed and the appearance of the larynx and mobility of the cords should be assessed. If there is any doubt as to whether there is fracture to the airway cartilage, a CT scan should be obtained. A fracture is more likely if there is an abnormal appearance of the larynx on nasendoscopy or if the vocal cords are not moving normally. A soft-tissue neck X-ray may also be useful for assessing prevertebral swelling, but if there is any doubt about the airway do not send the patient to an isolated X-ray department with only one unsupported radiographer in attendance.

Ingested foreign body

- These can be dangerous because if left they can cause perforation and mediastinitis. Chicken, lamb, beef or any other vertebrate bones are the most dangerous. The patient will usually be fairly definite about the history of swallow-ing a bone, and they can usually localise it pretty accurately if it is above the cricopharyngeus.

- Enquire about swallowing and examine the mouth, tonsils and base of the tongue carefully.

- Look for surgical emphysema.

- Obtain a lateral soft-tissue X-ray.

- Perform a flexible nasendoscopy looking for the foreign body and/or pooling of saliva.

- If the bone is visible on X-ray or there is gross swelling of the prevertebral tissues and the patient is dysphagic, they need endoscopy in theatre as soon as possible.

If the patient has swallowed a fish bone, they can be discharged with an appointment to return the next day for review if the following criteria are met:

- able to eat and drink normally
- no foreign body on X-ray (but many fish bones are radio-lucent)
- no prevertebral swelling on soft-tissue neck X-ray
- no pyrexia
- no surgical emphysema.

If they are no better the next day, they need endoscopy in theatre (ask them to come for review starved).

Food bolus obstruction

The history is of swallowing a large lump of food (it often seems to be steak!) which then gets stuck. The patient often has absolute dysphagia and is spitting out their own saliva. Take a careful history and really press the patient on whether there might be a bone present in the bolus. Enquire about previous symptoms of dysphagia, heartburn, weight loss, etc., and obtain a lateral soft-tissue neck X-ray just in case. Give the patient 20 mg intravenous Buscopan (a muscle relaxant). This can be repeated after 30 minutes if necessary and then three times a day. You can also try to give them a fizzy drink. If the patient does not recover quickly after the Buscopan (it some-times works like magic!), admit them for intravenous fluids. If the patient has not settled by the next morning they will need an endoscopy and removal of the bolus. If the patient settles after the Buscopan and can prove to you that they can drink a glass of water, they can be discharged with advice on eating a soft diet for a short while. In any case, *every patient must have a barium swallow arranged and be followed up in clinic*, as they may have a stricture or early malignancy which contributed to the obstruction in the first instance. If the obstruction seems to be low in the chest (and some patients can feel this pretty accurately), we often refer them to gastroenterology for a flexible gastroscopy. Foreign bodies that are low down in the oesophagus can be more difficult and hazardous to remove by rigid endoscope than by flexible scope.

Tonsillitis

This is probably the commonest condition that we see in the ENT clinic. The history is of a sore throat and possibly earache. It has usually become worse over the previous few days, and the patient may not be able to eat and drink. If the patient cannot eat and drink and has had analgesia, they cannot go home.

Admit the patient and give them analgesia, intravenous fluids and antibiotics and possibly intravenous dexamethasone. The patient is not nil by mouth, and can eat and drink as tolerated. Send blood tests for a full blood count and Paul–Bunnell test, and if you suspect glandular fever, for liver function tests, too.

Box 3.1   Glandular fever

- This is caused by infection with Epstein–Barr virus.

- It tends to affect teenagers and young adults.

- It causes widespread lymphadenopathy and can cause enlargement of the liver and spleen.

- These patients often present to ENT surgeons with superimposed tonsillitis.

- There is bilateral tonsillitis with copious amounts of white slough on the tonsils. There is also widespread lymphadenopathy.

- Lab tests to confirm the diagnosis are the Paul–Bunnell or Monospot test.

- The patient must not be given ampicillin as this can cause a rash to develop all over the body.

- The patient is treated for tonsillitis but must be warned that they may get repeated episodes of sore throat and may feel exhausted for quite a long period after infection.

- The patient must also be warned to avoid contact sports, especially if there is evidence of organomegaly on examination.

- If the liver function tests are abnormal the patient must be followed up by the GP until they return to normal.

A note on choice of antibiotics should be made here. If the patient has not had antibiotics prior to presentation, simply give them Penicillin V, as most of this tonsillitis is caused by streptococci. If the patient has had penicillin prior to presentation, consider Augmentin. If there is a suggestion of peritonsillitis (swelling in the tonsillar bed pushing the affected tonsil to the midline) or quinsy (peritonsillar abscess), give a cephalosporin and metronidazole. We mentioned the 'tonsillitis' with apparently normal tonsils above.

If you see a peritonsillar swelling, you should aspirate it. Attach a needle to a syringe and insert the needle into the fullest part of the peritonsillar area at three points and draw

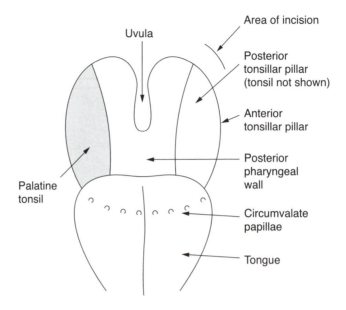

Uvula

Area of incision

Posterior
tonsillar pillar
(tonsil not shown)

Anterior
tonsillar pillar

Posterior
pharyngeal
wall

Palatine
tonsil

Circumvalate
papillae

Tongue

Figure 3.9 Area of incision.

back (*see* Figure 3.9). If you obtain pus, send it for culture. You can also use a guarded blade (a pointed blade with just the tip showing, the rest being 'guarded' with micropore tape wrapped several times around it) (*see* Figure 3.10).

Parapharyngeal abscess

This usually occurs as a consequence of tonsillitis, but it can occur in children after lymphadenitis. There is pain in the neck and torticollis. A swelling can be felt in the neck, which is very tender. The patient is pyrexial, is often drooling and has trismus. On examination of the mouth there is the appearance of a peritonsillar abscess (if you can see that far into the mouth!).

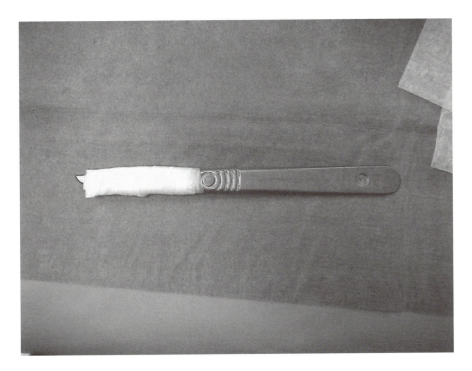

Figure 3.10 Guarded blade.

Assess the airway. If there is a suspicion of this condition, call someone senior and a CT scan will have to be requested. Admit the patient for intravenous antibiotics and give them nil by mouth. If the CT scan shows an abscess, the patient will need to go to theatre.

Neck abscess

This is a tender hot swelling that is fluctuant. *Do not be tempted to have a go with a knife under local anaesthetic in Accident and Emergency* – these abscesses are always deeper than you think! Remember to include travel history and TB exposure in the history. The patient should have a full examination, including flexible nasendoscopy. Admit them for intravenous antibiotics, and an ultrasound scan will help to make the decision on when to go to theatre. If the patient is admitted outside working hours, they can probably wait until the next morning.

Minimum dataset for recording the findings of flexible nasendoscopy

Introduction

Flexible nasendoscopy is performed regularly in the ENT clinic and is a very useful tool in diagnosing abnormalities of the upper aerodigestive tract. Nasendoscopy allows a view of many structures, but abnormalities can be missed if each area is not consciously inspected. In these days of increasing litigation it is important to comment on each area and a simple 'NAD' is probably not acceptable. We propose a minimum dataset for the recording of nasendoscopy findings which will aid communication between doctors and act as an aide-memoire for the doctor performing the procedure.

Fibreoptic flexible nasopharyngolaryngoscopy
Suggested minimum dataset

NOSE
Septum
Turbinates

NASOPHARYNX
Adenoidal pad
Eustachian tube orifice
Fossa of Rosen Muller

OROPHARYNX
Palate
Pillars
Lateral pharyngeal wall

HYPOPHARYNX
Tongue base
Vallecula
Epiglottis
Pyriform fossa

LARYNX
Anterior commissure
False folds
Vestibule
True folds
Posterior commissure
Arytenoids
Subglottis

Vocal cord movement

Source: Singh A and Lyons M (2004) Minimum dataset for the recording of findings of flexible nasopharyngolaryngoscopy. *J Laryngol Otol.* **118**(12): 972–3.

Discussion

Careful history taking and meticulous examination are the mainstays of all medicine and ENT is no exception. We are fortunate in having the tools to make a detailed examination of the upper aerodigestive tract without the need for sedation and general anaesthesia. Flexible nasendoscopy gives a huge amount of information about the anatomy and function of the structures inspected. Unfortunately, if each area is not inspected systematically valuable information can be lost. For more junior doctors a minimum dataset of questions (perhaps in the form of a stamp in the notes) will act to remind them to look at each area in turn. It will also help subsequent doctors to assess progress or deterioration in conditions. The recording of the data will not be too time-consuming and will lead to more thorough investigation of the patient which can only be of benefit.

Throat/head and neck operations

Tonsillectomy

The reasons for tonsillectomy can be categorised as absolute and relative. Absolute indications include removal for histological diagnosis of malignancy, and severe obstructive sleep apnoea (especially in children). Relative indications include recurrent tonsillitis, snoring and collection of tonsilloliths. The tonsils are removed through the mouth, so there are no cuts or stitches on the neck. The mucosa overlying the tonsillar bed is opened and the tonsil is 'peeled away' from its bed. The bleeding is stopped by means of ties or diathermy. The tonsillar bed is left open to heal by secondary intention, and it acts like a giant mouth ulcer. This is why the operation is so painful.

Risks of the procedure

- Pain and otalgia. This is a certainty rather than a risk. Tonsillectomy is a painful operation, and the pain is often worst on the fourth or fifth day (i.e. when the patient is at home!), after which it gets better. Analgesia should be taken regularly, even if the pain is not severe, for at least a week. The patient should also be encouraged to eat and drink as normally as possible, as this prevents stiffness developing in the pharyngeal muscles. Pain may also radiate to the ear. This does *not* mean that the patient has an ear infection – the pain is referred.

- Bleeding. As mentioned in the section on post-tonsillectomy bleeds, there are two risk periods (initially within the first 24 hours after operation, and then between 7 and 10 days after the operation). The figure quoted for the incidence of bleeding is 1–2%. This refers to bleeding that requires intervention (i.e. return to theatre or transfusion), but you will find more than this number come back having coughed up or spat out some blood.

- Appearance of the throat. It is important to warn the patient that there will be two large white patches where the tonsils used to be. This is normal and does not mean that there is infection.

Direct laryngopharyngooesophagoscopy (DL, DO, DP)

This involves examination of the upper aerodigestive tract using metal telescopes (*see* Figure 3.11).

Risks of the procedure

• Damage to teeth, bruising of lips, gums, etc. Metal telescopes are used to look round corners in order to gain access to the upper aerodigestive tract. Dental guards are used, but sometimes even with these precautions teeth can still be damaged. Always ask about caps/crowns, noting their

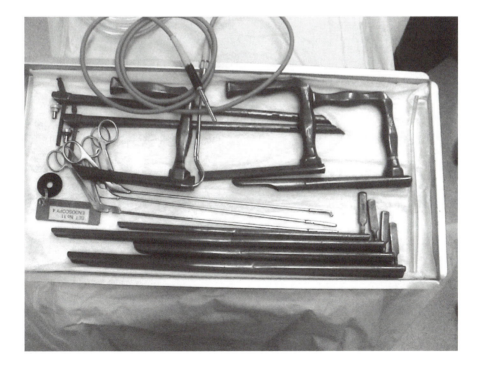

Figure 3.11   Metal telescopes.

presence and location, as capped teeth are not as strong as the patient's own.

- Sore throat. Most patients will have a sore throat after this procedure, both because they have been intubated and as a result of having the entire upper aerodigestive tract examined. This should settle quite quickly (certainly within a day or two, but usually within hours).

- Oesophageal perforation. This is a rare complication, but it is more common when oesophagoscopy is used to relieve bolus obstruction or remove a foreign body. You must tell the patient to report any chest or shoulder pain to the nursing staff immediately. Most of these perforations heal spontaneously. If there is a suspected perforation at operation, a nasogastric tube is placed under direct vision and the patient is given nil by mouth and kept on antibiotics for a few days before a contrast swallow is requested to make sure that there is healing.

- If the patient becomes clinically unwell, this will necessitate surgical intervention and closure of the perforation, which may involve cardiothoracic input. However, this is very unusual.

- Inability to remove a problematic foreign body. Most foreign bodies can be removed endoscopically. However, this sometimes proves too hazardous and the foreign body then has to be removed via the neck. This will necessitate the insertion of a nasogastric tube and giving the patient nil by mouth until the pharyngeal sutures have been shown to have healed (a contrast swallow will be necessary).

Thyroid surgery

This involves removing part or all of the thyroid gland. It is done for a variety of reasons, including suspected or known malignancy, an overactive thyroid gland that does not respond to medical treatment, and compressive symptoms caused by an enlarged thyroid gland.

The incision is on the front of the neck (*see* Figure 3.12) and goes past both sides of the midline (explain to the patient that this is for access). The surgeon always tries to put the incision in a skin crease. Usually the scar heals beautifully and is barely visible once it is fully healed.

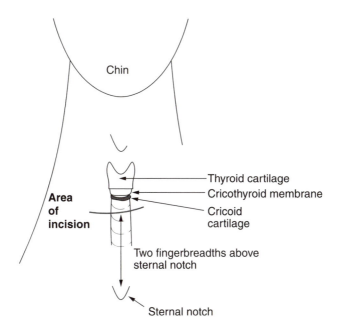

Figure 3.12 Incision for thyroid surgery.

Risks of the procedure

- Bleeding and drains. The thyroid is well supplied with blood vessels, and although the surgeon will try to ensure that the wound is completely dry before closure, reactionary haemorrhage can occur. A drain (or sometimes two) is inserted to collect any small amount of blood that is inevitably lost from the wound site after operation. It is removed as soon as it stops draining. *Note that a clip remover needs to be kept by the bed after a thyroid operation, and the clips should be removed along with internal stitches if a haematoma develops that is compromising the airway.*

- Low calcium level. The parathyroid glands are intimately related to the thyroid gland. Care is taken to identify and preserve them during surgery. This is sometimes not possible, or the blood supply to the parathyroid glands may become compromised. This leads to a drop in serum free calcium levels, which can be dangerous as it can lead to muscle spasm and cardiac instability. The patient must be instructed to inform the nursing staff if they notice any tingling around the mouth or in the fingers, or any spasms in the fingers. After total thyroidectomy, calcium levels are checked at 2 and 4 hours as a matter of routine. Warn the patient that they may need calcium supplements either temporarily or for life, especially if they are undergoing total thyroidectomy or completion thyroidectomy.

- Low thyroxine level. This usually only occurs if a total thyroidectomy or completion thyroidectomy is being performed. The patient will need thyroid hormone replacement for life.

- Recurrent laryngeal nerve damage. The recurrent laryngeal nerve is intimately related to the inferior thyroid artery. Surgeons now routinely seek the nerve and control the blood vessels and remove the gland while keeping the nerve in view. Some surgeons use a nerve monitor to warn them when they are coming close to the nerve. Even with these precautions neuropraxia can occur and cause temporary paralysis of the vocal cord. Bilateral vocal cord palsy can lead to airway compromise and necessitate a tracheostomy.

Box 3.2 Nerve monitor

These are increasingly used in ENT surgery during procedures that may cause damage to important nerves.

- For thyroid surgery an electrode is placed around the endotracheal tube at the point where it will lie between the vocal cords.

- Stimulation of the recurrent laryngeal nerve will cause movement of the vocal cords and will be detected by the electrode.

- The impulse is shown graphically on the monitor screen and also causes noise to be generated and this alerts the surgeon that he/she is close to the nerve. It is not a substitute for thorough anatomical knowledge but it can be a helpful reassurance.

- Further treatment/surgery. If the patient is undergoing a lobectomy for suspected cancer, then if cancer is proven a completion thyroidectomy may become necessary. If the patient is undergoing a total thyroidectomy for a known malignancy, further treatment (usually in the form of radioactive iodine) will be necessary.

Parathyroid surgery

The parathyroid glands are tiny glands, each about the size of a grain of rice, lying behind the thyroid gland. There are usually four, but there can be fewer or up to eight or nine. They produce parathyroid hormone which regulates calcium levels. Hypercalcaemia can occur if an adenoma develops in one gland (primary hyperparathyroidism) or if the patient has renal failure (tertiary hyperparathyroidism). For these reasons the parathyroid glands occasionally need to be removed. They are intimately related to the recurrent laryngeal nerves.

This operation is usually performed in order to relieve hypercalcaemia, and very rarely for parathyroid malignancy. If an adenoma is identified pre-operatively, only the affected gland is removed. If the patient suffers from renal failure, three out of four glands are removed and the fourth one is removed and implanted, possibly in the forearm. The incision is similar to that for thyroid surgery, except that it is usually shorter.

Most surgeons administer methylene blue before surgery. This stains the parathyroid glands, making them easier to identify. However, it also stains the skin, and the patient's relatives may find his or her grey appearance rather alarming post surgery! The urine will also be stained a blue/green colour for a few days afterwards.

Risks of the procedure

These are similar to the risks associated with thyroid surgery, with a few additional ones that are listed below.

- Inability to find all of the glands. Sometimes the parathyroid gland can descend into the chest during development and cannot be found during operation. Further scanning may be required.

- Hypocalcaemia. Calcium replacement may be necessary temporarily until an implanted parathyroid gland begins to function.

Parotidectomy

The parotid gland is a salivary gland that lies over the cheek, extending from the zygoma down to the angle of the jaw. Parotidectomy involves removal of the parotid gland, and 'parotidectomy' generally means superficial parotidectomy. The operation is most often performed to remove a lump in the parotid gland for histology, and for pleomorphic adenoma this is usually curative. Parotidectomy is also performed for chronic sialadenitis, although this is much less common.

The length of the incision that is used for this operation usually surprises the patient, as it is much longer than the lump that is to be removed. This incision is used to gain good exposure of the facial nerve, which is vital to a successful operation. The scar generally heals almost without trace, and you can console the patient by telling them that the incision is very like that made for a facelift!

Risks of the procedure

- Facial nerve damage. The five branches of this nerve run through the middle of the parotid gland. For this reason a long incision is made and the facial nerve is found and any tumour dissected off it. Most surgeons also now use a nerve monitor to alert them when they are coming close to the nerve. Damage to the facial nerve is still a risk. It is vital to demonstrate to the prospective patient what a facial palsy looks like, and to mention the fact that eye care will be needed if the worst happens and there is paralysis of the muscles that cause eye closure. For total parotidectomy for carcinoma of the parotid gland, the facial nerve will need to be sacrificed and the patient must be counselled about this. There are remedial procedures available in such cases (e.g. gold weights in the eyelids, facial hypoglossal transposition). Even when the nerve is intact at the end of the procedure, slight weakness may be apparent. This is only temporary, and the patient can be reassured that full function will be regained.

- Numbness around the ear. This occurs because the greater auricular nerve usually needs to be divided during the operation. The patch of numbness gets smaller with time, but there may be a permanent patch at the earlobe. Although apparently trivial, in the authors' experience it is the thing that patients complain about most, so it is vital to warn them about it beforehand.

- Frey's syndrome. This is the name for gustatory sweating, which occurs because the parasympathetic supply to the parotid gland is disrupted by the operation. It is thought that the parasympathetic supply instead then grows to the skin and causes sweating on the face when salivary flow is stimulated (e.g. by the sight or smell of food). It is quite a common phenomenon but does not prove bothersome to many patients. Treatments include scopolamine cream applied topically to the area, and division of the nerves in the tympanic plexus.

- Bleeding and drains. Once the superficial part of the parotid gland has been removed, a large 'raw' surface is left. This can bleed and cause a haematoma, or a seroma may be formed later. A drain is placed at the end of the operation, before closure, in order to reduce the 'dead space' between the flap and the raw edge of the remaining parotid gland.

- Scar. The reasons for the incision are mentioned above.

Submandibular duct stone removal and submandibular gland excision

The submandibular gland is a salivary gland that lies behind the ramus of the mandible and can be examined easily by bimanual palpation of the floor of the mouth. The examining fingers of one hand palpate the floor of the mouth (i.e. the fingers of one hand are inside the mouth) and the fingers of the other palpate the corresponding area of the neck. It produces saliva with a high mucus content and is therefore much more likely to form stones than the parotid gland, which produces more watery saliva.

If stones are palpable through the mouth then they can be removed perorally by placing a suture behind the stone to prevent it from moving back into the substance of the gland, and cutting down on to it. The duct is left open to heal by secondary intention.

The gland is usually removed because of recurrent stone formation and more rarely because of suspected malignancy. An incision is made at least two fingerbreadths below the mandible in order to preserve the marginal mandibular nerve, as this can loop below the mandible.

Risks of the procedure

- Nerve damage. Three nerves can be damaged during this procedure. The marginal mandibular part of the facial nerve has already been mentioned, and damage to this causes drooping of the corner of the mouth. The other two nerves are the hypoglossal nerve, damage to which causes paralysis of the affected side of the tongue, and the lingual nerve, which supplies common sensation to the anterior tongue and also carries special sense fibres (of taste) in its corda tympani component. These are all looked for and preserved during the operation.

- Bleeding and drains. As with most neck operations, haematoma and bleeding can occur and this is obviously undesirable in the neck, so a drain is used.

Summary of pre-admission requirements

4 Summary of pre-admission requirements

Now for the exciting part – your first pre-admission clinic! We remember desperately scribbling down the complications our registrar could remember before we went to the first clinic. This was not ideal, so as registrars we decided to formally write out what to tell the patient. We tried this out in St John's Hospital Chelmsford first, and it seemed to go down well. More and more units are now adopting a policy of consenting either by the surgeon listing the patient or the one actually doing the surgery. However, you may still be called upon to consent patients. If you are a career ENT SHO then you will have to learn to consent some day!

The purpose of the pre-admission clinic is to make sure that the patient is adequately prepared for theatre, and that any potential complications which may arise due to concomitant medical conditions are foreseen and if possible avoided. This is where your responsibility lies. You have done general medicine and surgery much more recently than your registrar and certainly than your consultant. A thorough history and examination are essential. If you have concerns about the medical state of the patient, get in touch with the anaesthetist concerned (you will find that they are much friendlier if they know about the condition in advance rather than having a nasty surprise on the day). However, you should use your common sense here, as not everyone with mild asthma needs referral for an anaesthetic opinion. A good trick is to determine exercise tolerance or whether the patient has ever been hospitalised for the condition. If you are lucky and have a sympathetic senior, any serious problems will have been picked up at the time of listing, and the listing surgeon will have sent the patient for a specialist opinion. Make sure that the letters and investigations are in the notes (phone the relevant secretary to find out whether this is the case).

The investigations that you need to do can vary from one hospital to another, and most hospitals have a policy on what blood tests and/or X-rays need to be obtained. Bear in mind that you probably won't be criticised too harshly for over-enthusiastic requesting of tests (within reason), but you will certainly make yourself very unpopular if you don't do adequate investigations.

General investigations undertaken for any patient undergoing surgery

- **Full blood count (FBC):** Women of childbearing age (this is not true in all units, check with yours), any cancer surgery, moderate to severe blood loss predicted, suspected anaemia, suspected malnourishment, the elderly.

- **Sickle-cell tests:** Some anaesthetists want sickle-cell tests to be performed on everyone (this is rare, and you may have to accept being told off by an anaesthetist on the first day if they want this). In general only patients of Afro-Caribbean and Asian origin need a sickle-cell test.

- **Urea and electrolytes (U&E):** The elderly, hypertensive patients or those on antihypertensive medication (especially

ACE inhibitors or diuretics), diabetics, history of renal disease, surgery predicted to be long and complex, suspected dehydration.

- **Liver function tests (LFTs):** Suspected alcohol abuse, obvious bruising on the patient, cancer surgery (specifically to look for albumin levels), suspected malnutrition, previous history of liver disease.

- **Clotting:** Suspected alcohol abuse, obvious bruising, patients on anticoagulants (get advice from haematology on when and how to stop medication, whether the patient needs heparinisation, etc.), moderate to severe blood loss predicted as a consequence of surgery, known liver disease.

- **Glucose:** Known or suspected diabetics (consider HbA_{1C}).

- **Blood gases:** Moderate to severe asthma/chronic obstructive airways disease, known chest condition, request from anaesthetist. In some units respiratory function tests are also required.

- **Group and save/cross-matching:** It is very difficult to generalise here. The best advice is to ask your consultant or registrar. Obviously if the patient is going to undergo major head and neck surgery they will need saved units (the exact number will be decided by the surgeon). It is often better to err on the side of caution and to group and save the patient at a minimum. If you are in doubt, ask your senior.

- **ECG:** Patients with known cardiac history, hypertensive patients (even when on treatment), cancer patients (most head and neck cancer patients smoke), diabetics. Some units advocate anyone over 60 years of age.

- **Chest X-ray (CXR):** Many units will ask you to justify your request, and age alone is no longer a good justification. Known chest disease (asthma, chronic obstructive airways disease), known heart disease, cancer surgery (to look for chest metastases), abnormal results on chest examination, thyroid surgery (will allow assessment of deviation of the trachea).

Also make sure that you take time to read the notes carefully (we know that pre-admission is sometimes very busy, but this is not an adequate excuse when the scans, etc. are not present). If a scan or other investigation has been requested in the past, make sure that you ask the pre-admission staff to find films, etc. No scans often mean no operation, and neither the patient nor the surgeon will thank you if this happens.

As a general rule the operations listed below will need the investigations indicated. However, you should always read the notes, as there are occasionally surprises!

- **Functional endoscopic sinus surgery (FESS):** Scans are always needed. Not all polypectomies will have had scans.

- **Mastoid operations:** These patients may or may not have had CT scans, so check the notes.

- **Parotid and submandibular glands:** These patients will have had ultrasound examination and possibly fine needle aspiration (FNA), so check the notes. A written report of the FNA should be in the notes before surgery.

- **Any head and neck cancer cases:** These will probably have had scans and biopsies. Make sure that the histology report is in the notes before surgery.

- **DL/DO/DP:** These cases may have had a barium swallow.

- **Pharyngeal pouch cases:** These will always have had a barium swallow.

- **Cosmetic operations (e.g. rhinoplasty or pinnaplasty):** These cases need photographs.

Useful books and websites

- www.entuk.org. The patient information part gives a good summary of how operations are performed and the potential complications.

- Scott-Brown V (1997) *Otolaryngology* (6e). Butterworth Heinemann, London. This is useful for reference and in-depth reading, but is probably a bit heavy when you are on call.

- Bleach N, Milford C and Van Hasselt A (eds) (1997) *Operative Otorhinolaryngology*. Blackwell Science, London. This is excellent for reading before a theatre session, as it gives a step-by-step account of how operations are performed as well as providing information about complications, etc.

- Carlisle J, Langham J and Thoms G (2004) Editorial I: Guidelines for routine pre-operative testing. *Br J Anaest.* **93**: 495–7. This provides guidelines on elective patient laboratory tests.

Glossary

As with most specialities, ENT has a language all of its own. Below is a glossary of terms that may not be familiar to non-ENT practitioners.

- **Abducens nucleus** Nucleus of the sixth cranial nerve. It lies in the pons and the facial nerve loops around it.

- **Aditus ad antrum 'hallway'** The area leading from the mastoid into the middle ear.

- **Audiogram** Hearing test. Ideally the patient is in a sound-proofed booth and asked to wear headphones. Monotonal (and therefore unifrequency tones) sounds are played to the patient, who is asked to indicate when the tone is heard. A threshold sound level is found for each frequency and plotted on a graph.

- **Auroscope** Device for examining the outer ear canal and eardrum. The viewing aperture is through the light, and this prevents the examiner's head from blocking the illumination of the ear canal.

- **BIPP** Bismuth iodoform paraffin paste, an antiseptic substance in which ribbon gauze is soaked for nasal and ear dressings.

- **Cahart's notch** Occurs with otosclerosis where the conductive and sensorineural parts of the audiogram come closer together at 2000 Hz.

- **Cauliflower ear** Name given to the deformed pinna cartilage that develops when its blood supply has been compromised (usually by a pinna haematoma). The pinna loses its normal contours, becomes thicker and can collapse.

- **Cholesteatoma** Collection of squamous epithelium in the middle ear and mastoid air-cell system. It may be congenital or acquired, and it leads to repeated infection and destruction of middle ear structures.

- **Corda tympani** Component of the facial nerve (but actually arising and travelling with the nervus intermedius for part of its length) that contains taste fibres for the anterior two-thirds of the tongue. It is given off shortly before the facial nerve enters the stylomastoid foramen, and crosses the middle ear in close contact with the eardrum and the neck of the malleus.

- **CVA** Cerebrovascular accident or stroke.

- **Eardrum** Medial border of the outer ear canal and lateral border of the middle ear. It consists of two areas, namely the pars tensa (which is formed from three layers of tissue) and the pars flaccida (which consists of only two layers).

- **Facial nerve** Seventh cranial nerve. Its main function is to supply the muscles of facial expression. It also has sensory, special sense (taste) and secretomotor fibres. It is intimately related to the middle and inner ear.

- **Geniculate ganglion** Lies at the first bend of the facial nerve. The greater petrosal nerve is given off at this point to eventually supply the lacrimal gland.

- **Genu** Literally means 'knee'.

- **Haemotympanum** Blood behind the eardrum, usually as a result of trauma (skull fracture).

- **Helix** Outer fold of pinna cartilage.

- **Incus** Also known as the 'anvil', the second bone of hearing. It articulates with the malleus and can sometimes be seen on examination of the ear canal.

- **Internal auditory meatus** The facial nerve exits the cranial cavity here and enters the petrous temporal bone.

- **Lateral semicircular canal** The semicircular canals are fluid-filled canals which have sensory cells that detect angular acceleration of the head.

- **Lingual nerve** Nerve that supplies the oral part of the tongue. It has a trigeminal component which supplies common sensation, a corda tympani component which carries the taste fibres, and a secretomotor component which supplies the anterior lingual gland.

- **Malleus** Also known as the 'hammer', the largest bone of hearing. It is usually visible on examination of the outer ear canal as it is attached to the medial surface of the eardrum. It has a head, neck and handle, and it articulates with the incus.

- **Mastoiditis** Inflammation of the mucosa of the mastoid air-cell system.

- **Myringoplasty** Repair of a tympanic membrane perforation using a graft.

- **Nervus intermedius** Component of the facial nerve that supplies the secretomotor, special sense and sensory parts of the nerve supply.

- **Nystagmus** A combination of alternating slow and fast saccadic eye movements in opposite directions.

- **Otitis externa** Inflammation of the external ear canal. It is usually due to bacterial infection (acutely caused by streptococci and staphylococci, or chronically caused by Gram-negative organisms and fungi).

- **Otitis media** Inflammation of the middle ear. It can be acute (more usual in children) or chronic.

- **Parotid gland** Paired salivary gland producing serous secretions containing little calcium. It lies on the lateral side of the face in front of the ear canal and superficial to the ramus of the mandible.

- **Pars flaccida** Part of the eardrum above the head of the malleus. It can become retracted, and cholesteatoma usually forms behind this area.

- **Permeatally** Through the ear canal. This usually refers to myringoplasties and stapedectomies.

- **Pinnaplasty** Correction of prominent or 'bat' ears by formation of a helical fold in the pinna.

- **Pons** Part of the brainstem.

- **Promontory** Bulge in the medial wall of the middle ear. It lies antero-inferiorly, and represents the basal turn of the cochlea.

- **Rhinorrhoea** Nasal discharge. It usually refers to anterior rhinorrhoea, whereas posterior rhinorrhoea is usually referred to as postnasal drip.

- **Rinne's test** Test of hearing to determine whether conduction is better through air or bone. A tuning fork is struck (512 Hz or 1024 Hz) and placed on the mastoid bone. The patient is then asked to indicate whether a tone is heard and also to indicate when it disappears. Once the tone has disappeared the tuning fork is placed about 2–3 cm from the aperture of the outer ear canal. The patient should be able to hear the tone again if the hearing in that ear is normal.

- **Spine of sphenoid** Posterior end of the medial part of the greater wing of the sphenoid. Its base is perforated by the foramen spinosum for the middle meningeal vessels.

- **Stylomastoid foramen** Exit point of the facial nerve from the skull.

- **Tinnitus** Perception of sound when there is no obvious outside stimulus. It can be subjective or objective.

- **Tympanogram** Test of compliance of the eardrum.

- **Tympanic plexus** Plexus of nerves consisting mainly of the tympanic branch of the glossopharyngeal nerve. It lies on the promontory and here is joined by sympathetic fibres from the internal carotid nerve. The nerves from the plexus supply sensory and vasomotor fibres to the mucous membranes of the tympanic cavity and the Eustachian tube.

- **Vertigo** Defined as an illusion of movement, not just rotation.

- **Vestibulocochlear nerve** Eighth cranial nerve, responsible for conveying impulses associated with hearing and balance.

- **Vibrissae** Hairs lining the inside of the nose, which trap contaminants and allow the filtration of inspired air.

- **Weber's test** Test of hearing to determine whether the hearing on one side is better than that on the other. A tuning fork is struck and its base is placed in the midline on the forehead (it can also be placed on the teeth). The patient is asked to indicate whether they can hear the tone and from where it appears to arise. In normal symmetrical hearing the tone should appear to be coming from the midline.

Index

Page numbers in *italics* refer to figures.